THE OFFICIAL PARENT'S SOURCEBOOK

on

NIEMANN-PICK DISEASE

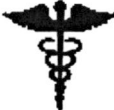

JAMES N. PARKER, M.D.
AND PHILIP M. PARKER, PH.D., EDITORS

ICON Health Publications
ICON Group International, Inc.
4370 La Jolla Village Drive, 4th Floor
San Diego, CA 92122 USA

Copyright ©2002 by ICON Group International, Inc.

Copyright ©2002 by ICON Group International, Inc. All rights reserved. This book is protected by copyright. No part of it may be reproduced, stored in a retrieval system, or transmitted in any form or by any means, electronic, mechanical, photocopying, recording or otherwise, without written permission from the publisher.

Printed in the United States of America.

Last digit indicates print number: 10 9 8 7 6 4 5 3 2 1

Publisher, Health Care: Tiffany LaRochelle
Editor(s): James Parker, M.D., Philip Parker, Ph.D.

Publisher's note: The ideas, procedures, and suggestions contained in this book are not intended as a substitute for consultation with your child's physician. All matters regarding your child's health require medical supervision. As new medical or scientific information becomes available from academic and clinical research, recommended treatments and drug therapies may undergo changes. The authors, editors, and publisher have attempted to make the information in this book up to date and accurate in accord with accepted standards at the time of publication. The authors, editors, and publisher are not responsible for errors or omissions or for consequences from application of the book, and make no warranty, expressed or implied, in regard to the contents of this book. Any practice described in this book should be applied by the reader in accordance with professional standards of care used in regard to the unique circumstances that may apply in each situation, in close consultation with a qualified physician. The reader is advised to always check product information (package inserts) for changes and new information regarding dose and contraindications before administering any drug or pharmacological product. Caution is especially urged when using new or infrequently ordered drugs, herbal remedies, vitamins and supplements, alternative therapies, complementary therapies and medicines, and integrative medical treatments.

Cataloging-in-Publication Data

Parker, James N., 1961-
Parker, Philip M., 1960-

The Official Parent's Sourcebook on Niemann-Pick Disease: A Revised and Updated Directory for the Internet Age/James N. Parker and Philip M. Parker, editors
  p.   cm.
Includes bibliographical references, glossary and index.
ISBN: 0-597-83025-8
  1. Niemann-Pick Disease-Popular works.   I. Title.

BRIDGEND LIBRARY & INFORMATION SERVICE	
Bertrams	27.02.08
616.39	£22.95

Disclaimer

This publication is not intended to be used for the diagnosis or treatment of a health problem or as a substitute for consultation with licensed medical professionals. It is sold with the understanding that the publisher, editors, and authors are not engaging in the rendering of medical, psychological, financial, legal, or other professional services.

References to any entity, product, service, or source of information that may be contained in this publication should not be considered an endorsement, either direct or implied, by the publisher, editors, or authors. ICON Group International, Inc., the editors, or the authors are not responsible for the content of any Web pages nor publications referenced in this publication.

Copyright Notice

If a physician wishes to copy limited passages from this sourcebook for parent use, this right is automatically granted without written permission from ICON Group International, Inc. (ICON Group). However, all of ICON Group publications are copyrighted. With exception to the above, copying our publications in whole or in part, for whatever reason, is a violation of copyright laws and can lead to penalties and fines. Should you want to copy tables, graphs or other materials, please contact us to request permission (e-mail: iconedit@san.rr.com). ICON Group often grants permission for very limited reproduction of our publications for internal use, press releases, and academic research. Such reproduction requires confirmed permission from ICON Group International Inc. **The disclaimer above must accompany all reproductions, in whole or in part, of this sourcebook.**

Dedication

To the healthcare professionals dedicating their time and efforts to the study of Niemann-Pick disease.

Acknowledgements

The collective knowledge generated from academic and applied research summarized in various references has been critical in the creation of this sourcebook which is best viewed as a comprehensive compilation and collection of information prepared by various official agencies which directly or indirectly are dedicated to Niemann-Pick disease. All of the *Official Parent's Sourcebooks* draw from various agencies and institutions associated with the United States Department of Health and Human Services, and in particular, the Office of the Secretary of Health and Human Services (OS), the Administration for Children and Families (ACF), the Administration on Aging (AOA), the Agency for Healthcare Research and Quality (AHRQ), the Agency for Toxic Substances and Disease Registry (ATSDR), the Centers for Disease Control and Prevention (CDC), the Food and Drug Administration (FDA), the Healthcare Financing Administration (HCFA), the Health Resources and Services Administration (HRSA), the Indian Health Service (IHS), the institutions of the National Institutes of Health (NIH), the Program Support Center (PSC), and the Substance Abuse and Mental Health Services Administration (SAMHSA). In addition to these sources, information gathered from the National Library of Medicine, the United States Patent Office, the European Union, and their related organizations has been invaluable in the creation of this sourcebook. Some of the work represented was financially supported by the Research and Development Committee at INSEAD. This support is gratefully acknowledged. Finally, special thanks are owed to Tiffany LaRochelle for her excellent editorial support.

About the Editors

James N. Parker, M.D.

Dr. James N. Parker received his Bachelor of Science degree in Psychobiology from the University of California, Riverside and his M.D. from the University of California, San Diego. In addition to authoring numerous research publications, he has lectured at various academic institutions. Dr. Parker is the medical editor for the *Official Parent's Sourcebook* series published by ICON Health Publications.

Philip M. Parker, Ph.D.

Philip M. Parker is the Eli Lilly Chair Professor of Innovation, Business and Society at INSEAD (Fontainebleau, France and Singapore). Dr. Parker has also been Professor at the University of California, San Diego and has taught courses at Harvard University, the Hong Kong University of Science and Technology, the Massachusetts Institute of Technology, Stanford University, and UCLA. Dr. Parker is the associate editor for the *Official Parent's Sourcebook* series published by ICON Health Publications.

About ICON Health Publications

In addition to Niemann-Pick disease, *Official Parent's Sourcebooks* are available for the following related topics:

- The Official Patient's Sourcebook on Fabry
- The Official Patient's Sourcebook on Gaucher
- The Official Patient's Sourcebook on Leigh's Disease
- The Official Patient's Sourcebook on Lesch Nyham
- The Official Patient's Sourcebook on Menkes Disease
- The Official Patient's Sourcebook on Metachromatic Leukodystrophy
- The Official Patient's Sourcebook on Mucopolysaccharidoses
- The Official Patient's Sourcebook on Pelizaeus Merzbacher
- The Official Patient's Sourcebook on Refsum Disease
- The Official Patient's Sourcebook on Sandhoff Disease
- The Official Patient's Sourcebook on Schilder's Disease
- The Official Patient's Sourcebook on Split Up Leukodystrophy
- The Official Patient's Sourcebook on Tay Sachs

To discover more about ICON Health Publications, simply check with your preferred online booksellers, including Barnes & Noble.com and Amazon.com which currently carry all of our titles. Or, feel free to contact us directly for bulk purchases or institutional discounts:

ICON Group International, Inc.
4370 La Jolla Village Drive, Fourth Floor
San Diego, CA 92122 USA
Fax: 858-546-4341
Web site: **www.icongrouponline.com/health**

Table of Contents

INTRODUCTION 1
   Overview 1
   Organization 3
   Scope 3
   Moving Forward 4

PART I: THE ESSENTIALS 7

CHAPTER 1. THE ESSENTIALS ON NIEMANN-PICK DISEASE: GUIDELINES 9
   Overview 9
   What Is Niemann-Pick Disease? 10
   Is There Any Treatment? 11
   What Is the Prognosis? 11
   What Research Is Being Done? 12
   For More Information 12
   More Guideline Sources 13
   Vocabulary Builder 15

CHAPTER 2. SEEKING GUIDANCE 17
   Overview 17
   Associations and Niemann-Pick Disease 17
   Finding More Associations 24
   Finding Doctors 25
   Finding a Neurologist 26
   Selecting Your Doctor 27
   Working with Your Child's Doctor 27
   Broader Health-Related Resources 28
   Vocabulary Builder 28

CHAPTER 3. CLINICAL TRIALS AND NIEMANN-PICK DISEASE 31
   Overview 31
   Recent Trials on Niemann-Pick Disease 34
   Benefits and Risks 35
   Keeping Current on Clinical Trials 38
   General References 39
   Vocabulary Builder 40

PART II: ADDITIONAL RESOURCES AND ADVANCED MATERIAL 41

CHAPTER 4. STUDIES ON NIEMANN-PICK DISEASE 43
   Overview 43
   Federally-Funded Research on Niemann-Pick Disease 43
   E-Journals: PubMed Central 58

viii Contents

    The National Library of Medicine: PubMed 60
    Vocabulary Builder 60
  CHAPTER 5. BOOKS ON NIEMANN-PICK DISEASE 67
    Overview 67
    Book Summaries: Online Booksellers 67
    The National Library of Medicine Book Index 67
    Chapters on Niemann-Pick Disease 68
    General Home References 69

PART III. APPENDICES 71

  APPENDIX A. RESEARCHING YOUR CHILD'S MEDICATIONS 73
    Overview 73
    Your Child's Medications: The Basics 73
    Learning More about Your Child's Medications 75
    Commercial Databases 76
    Contraindications and Interactions (Hidden Dangers) 77
    A Final Warning 78
    General References 79
  APPENDIX B. RESEARCHING NUTRITION 81
    Overview 81
    Food and Nutrition: General Principles 82
    Finding Studies on Niemann-Pick Disease 86
    Federal Resources on Nutrition 90
    Additional Web Resources 91
  APPENDIX C. FINDING MEDICAL LIBRARIES 93
    Overview 93
    Preparation 93
    Finding a Local Medical Library 94
    Medical Libraries Open to the Public 94
  APPENDIX D. YOUR CHILD'S RIGHTS AND INSURANCE 101
    Overview 101
    Your Child's Rights as a Patient 101
    Parent Responsibilities 105
    Choosing an Insurance Plan 106
    Medicaid 108
    NORD's Medication Assistance Programs 108
    Additional Resources 109
    Vocabulary Builder 110

ONLINE GLOSSARIES 113

    Online Dictionary Directories 114

NIEMANN-PICK DISEASE GLOSSARY 115

General Dictionaries and Glossaries *123*
INDEX **125**

INTRODUCTION

Overview

Dr. C. Everett Koop, former U.S. Surgeon General, once said, "The best prescription is knowledge."[1] The Agency for Healthcare Research and Quality (AHRQ) of the National Institutes of Health (NIH) echoes this view and recommends that all parents incorporate education into the treatment process. According to the AHRQ:

> Finding out more about your [child's] condition is a good place to start. By contacting groups that support your [child's] condition, visiting your local library, and searching on the Internet, you can find good information to help guide your decisions for your [child's] treatment. Some information may be hard to find—especially if you don't know where to look.[2]

As the AHRQ mentions, finding the right information is not an obvious task. Though many physicians and public officials had thought that the emergence of the Internet would do much to assist parents in obtaining reliable information, in March 2001 the National Institutes of Health issued the following warning:

> The number of Web sites offering health-related resources grows every day. Many sites provide valuable information, while others may have information that is unreliable or misleading.[3]

---

[1] Quotation from http://www.drkoop.com.
[2] The Agency for Healthcare Research and Quality (AHRQ): http://www.ahcpr.gov/consumer/diaginfo.htm.
[3] From the NIH, National Cancer Institute (NCI): **http://cancertrials.nci.nih.gov/beyond/evaluating.html**.

Since the late 1990s, physicians have seen a general increase in parent Internet usage rates. Parents frequently enter their children's doctor's offices with printed Web pages of home remedies in the guise of latest medical research. This scenario is so common that doctors often spend more time dispelling misleading information than guiding children through sound therapies. *The Official Parent's Sourcebook on Niemann-Pick Disease* has been created for parents who have decided to make education and research an integral part of the treatment process. The pages that follow will tell you where and how to look for information covering virtually all topics related to Niemann-Pick disease, from the essentials to the most advanced areas of research.

The title of this book includes the word "official." This reflects the fact that the sourcebook draws from public, academic, government, and peer-reviewed research. Selected readings from various agencies are reproduced to give you some of the latest official information available to date on Niemann-Pick disease.

Given parents' increasing sophistication in using the Internet, abundant references to reliable Internet-based resources are provided throughout this sourcebook. Where possible, guidance is provided on how to obtain free-of-charge, primary research results as well as more detailed information via the Internet. E-book and electronic versions of this sourcebook are fully interactive with each of the Internet sites mentioned (clicking on a hyperlink automatically opens your browser to the site indicated). Hard copy users of this sourcebook can type cited Web addresses directly into their browsers to obtain access to the corresponding sites. Since we are working with ICON Health Publications, hard copy *Sourcebooks* are frequently updated and printed on demand to ensure that the information provided is current.

In addition to extensive references accessible via the Internet, every chapter presents a "Vocabulary Builder." Many health guides offer glossaries of technical or uncommon terms in an appendix. In editing this sourcebook, we have decided to place a smaller glossary within each chapter that covers terms used in that chapter. Given the technical nature of some chapters, you may need to revisit many sections. Building one's vocabulary of medical terms in such a gradual manner has been shown to improve the learning process.

We must emphasize that no sourcebook on Niemann-Pick disease should affirm that a specific diagnostic procedure or treatment discussed in a research study, patent, or doctoral dissertation is "correct" or your child's best option. This sourcebook is no exception. Each child is unique. Deciding on appropriate options is always up to parents in consultation with their children's physicians and healthcare providers.

Organization

This sourcebook is organized into three parts. Part I explores basic techniques to researching Niemann-Pick disease (e.g. finding guidelines on diagnosis, treatments, and prognosis), followed by a number of topics, including information on how to get in touch with organizations, associations, or other parent networks dedicated to Niemann-Pick disease. It also gives you sources of information that can help you find a doctor in your local area specializing in treating Niemann-Pick disease. Collectively, the material presented in Part I is a complete primer on basic research topics for Niemann-Pick disease.

Part II moves on to advanced research dedicated to Niemann-Pick disease. Part II is intended for those willing to invest many hours of hard work and study. It is here that we direct you to the latest scientific and applied research on Niemann-Pick disease. When possible, contact names, links via the Internet, and summaries are provided. It is in Part II where the vocabulary process becomes important as authors publishing advanced research frequently use highly specialized language. In general, every attempt is made to recommend "free-to-use" options.

Part III provides appendices of useful background reading covering Niemann-Pick disease or related disorders. The appendices are dedicated to more pragmatic issues facing parents. Accessing materials via medical libraries may be the only option for some parents, so a guide is provided for finding local medical libraries which are open to the public. Part III, therefore, focuses on advice that goes beyond the biological and scientific issues facing children with Niemann-Pick disease and their families.

Scope

While this sourcebook covers Niemann-Pick disease, doctors, research publications, and specialists may refer to your child's condition using a variety of terms. Therefore, you should understand that Niemann-Pick disease is often considered a synonym or a condition closely related to the following:

- Lipid Histiocytosis

- Lipidosis, Sphingomyelin
- Sphingomyelin Lipidosis
- Sphingomyelinase Deficiency

In addition to synonyms and related conditions, physicians may refer to Niemann-Pick disease using certain coding systems. The International Classification of Diseases, 9th Revision, Clinical Modification (ICD-9-CM) is the most commonly used system of classification for the world's illnesses. Your physician may use this coding system as an administrative or tracking tool. The following classification is commonly used for Niemann-Pick disease:[4]

- 272.7 niemann-pick disease

For the purposes of this sourcebook, we have attempted to be as inclusive as possible, looking for official information for all of the synonyms relevant to Niemann-Pick disease. You may find it useful to refer to synonyms when accessing databases or interacting with healthcare professionals and medical librarians.

Moving Forward

Since the 1980s, the world has seen a proliferation of healthcare guides covering most illnesses. Some are written by parents, patients, or their family members. These generally take a layperson's approach to understanding and coping with an illness or disorder. They can be uplifting, encouraging, and highly supportive. Other guides are authored by physicians or other healthcare providers who have a more clinical outlook. Each of these two styles of guide has its purpose and can be quite useful.

As editors, we have chosen a third route. We have chosen to expose you to as many sources of official and peer-reviewed information as practical, for the purpose of educating you about basic and advanced knowledge as recognized by medical science today. You can think of this sourcebook as your personal Internet age reference librarian.

---

[4] This list is based on the official version of the World Health Organization's 9th Revision, International Classification of Diseases (ICD-9). According to the National Technical Information Service, "ICD-9CM extensions, interpretations, modifications, addenda, or errata other than those approved by the U.S. Public Health Service and the Health Care Financing Administration are not to be considered official and should not be utilized. Continuous maintenance of the ICD-9-CM is the responsibility of the federal government."

Why "Internet age"? When their child has been diagnosed with Niemann-Pick disease, parents will often log on to the Internet, type words into a search engine, and receive several Web site listings which are mostly irrelevant or redundant. Parents are left to wonder where the relevant information is, and how to obtain it. Since only the smallest fraction of information dealing with Niemann-Pick disease is even indexed in search engines, a non-systematic approach often leads to frustration and disappointment. With this sourcebook, we hope to direct you to the information you need that you would not likely find using popular Web directories. Beyond Web listings, in many cases we will reproduce brief summaries or abstracts of available reference materials. These abstracts often contain distilled information on topics of discussion.

Before beginning your search for information, it is important for you to realize that Niemann-Pick disease is considered a relatively uncommon condition. Because of this, far less research is conducted on Niemann-Pick disease compared to other health problems afflicting larger populations, like breast cancer or heart disease. Nevertheless, this sourcebook will prove useful for two reasons. First, if more information does become available on Niemann-Pick disease, the sources given in this book will be the most likely to report or make such information available. Second, some will find it important to know about patient support, symptom management, or diagnostic procedures that may be relevant to both Niemann-Pick disease and other conditions. By using the sources listed in the following chapters, self-directed research can be conducted on broader topics that are related to Niemann-Pick disease but not readily uncovered using general Internet search engines (e.g. www.google.com or www.yahoo.com). In this way, we have designed this sourcebook to complement these general search engines that can provide useful information and access to online patient support groups.[5]

---

[5] For example, one can simply go to **www.google.com**, or other general search engines (e.g. **www.yahoo.com**, **www.aol.com**, **www.msn.com**) and type in "Niemann-Pick disease support group" to find any active online support groups dedicated to Niemann-Pick disease.

While we focus on the more scientific aspects of Niemann-Pick disease, there is, of course, the emotional side to consider. Later in the sourcebook, we provide a chapter dedicated to helping you find parent groups and associations that can provide additional support beyond research produced by medical science. We hope that the choices we have made give you and your child the most options in moving forward. In this way, we wish you the best in your efforts to incorporate this educational approach into your child's treatment plan.

The Editors

PART I: THE ESSENTIALS

ABOUT PART I

Part I has been edited to give you access to what we feel are "the essentials" on Niemann-Pick disease. The essentials typically include a definition or description of the condition, a discussion of who it affects, the signs or symptoms, tests or diagnostic procedures, and treatments for disease. Your child's doctor or healthcare provider may have already explained the essentials of Niemann-Pick disease to you or even given you a pamphlet or brochure describing the condition. Now you are searching for more in-depth information. As editors, we have decided, nevertheless, to include a discussion on where to find essential information that can complement what the doctor has already told you. In this section we recommend a process, not a particular Web site or reference book. The process ensures that, as you search the Web, you gain background information in such a way as to maximize your understanding.

CHAPTER 1. THE ESSENTIALS ON NIEMANN-PICK DISEASE: GUIDELINES

Overview

Official agencies, as well as federally-funded institutions supported by national grants, frequently publish a variety of guidelines on Niemann-Pick disease. These are typically called "Fact Sheets" or "Guidelines." They can take the form of a brochure, information kit, pamphlet, or flyer. Often they are only a few pages in length. The great advantage of guidelines over other sources is that they are often written with the parent in mind. Since new guidelines on Niemann-Pick disease can appear at any moment and be published by a number of sources, the best approach to finding guidelines is to systematically scan the Internet-based services that post them.

The National Institutes of Health (NIH)[6]

The National Institutes of Health (NIH) is the first place to search for relatively current guidelines and fact sheets on Niemann-Pick disease. Originally founded in 1887, the NIH is one of the world's foremost medical research centers and the federal focal point for medical research in the United States. At any given time, the NIH supports some 35,000 research grants at universities, medical schools, and other research and training institutions, both nationally and internationally. The rosters of those who have conducted research or who have received NIH support over the years include the world's most illustrious scientists and physicians. Among them are 97 scientists who have won the Nobel Prize for achievement in medicine.

---

[6] Adapted from the NIH: **http://www.nih.gov/about/NIHoverview.html**.

There is no guarantee that any one Institute will have a guideline on a specific medical condition, though the National Institutes of Health collectively publish over 600 guidelines for both common and rare disorders. The best way to access NIH guidelines is via the Internet. Although the NIH is organized into many different Institutes and Offices, the following is a list of key Web sites where you are most likely to find NIH clinical guidelines and publications dealing with Niemann-Pick disease and associated conditions:

- Office of the Director (OD); guidelines consolidated across agencies available at **http://www.nih.gov/health/consumer/conkey.htm**
- National Library of Medicine (NLM); extensive encyclopedia (A.D.A.M., Inc.) with guidelines available at **http://www.nlm.nih.gov/medlineplus/healthtopics.html**
- National Institute of Neurological Disorders and Stroke (NINDS); **http://www.ninds.nih.gov/health_and_medical/disorder_index.htm**

Among the above, the National Institute of Neurological Disorders and Stroke (NINDS) is particularly noteworthy. The mission of the NINDS is to reduce the burden of neurological disease—a burden borne by every age group, by every segment of society, by people all over the world.[7] To support this mission, the NINDS conducts, fosters, coordinates, and guides research on the causes, prevention, diagnosis, and treatment of neurological disorders and stroke, and supports basic research in related scientific areas. The following patient guideline was recently published by the NINDS on Niemann-Pick disease.

What Is Niemann-Pick Disease?[8]

Niemann-Pick disease (NP) is an inherited metabolic disorder in which harmful quantities of a fatty substance accumulate in the spleen, liver, lungs, bone marrow, and, in some patients, the brain. The clinical designations applied to NP are somewhat erratic. Patients are currently subdivided into 4 categories. In the first, called type A, enlargement of the liver and spleen are apparent in infancy and profound brain damage is evident. These children rarely live beyond 18 months. In the second group, called type B,

---

[7] This paragraph has been adapted from the NINDS: **http://www.ninds.nih.gov/about_ninds/mission.htm**. "Adapted" signifies that a passage has been reproduced exactly or slightly edited for this book.

[8] Adapted from The National Institute of Neurological Disorders and Stroke (NINDS): **http://www.ninds.nih.gov/health_and_medical/disorders/niemann.doc.htm**.

enlargement of the liver and spleen characteristically occur in the pre-teen years. Most of these patients also have pulmonary difficulties, but the brain is not affected. The fatty material that accumulates in types A and B is called sphingomyelin. This lipid is a major component of the membrane of all cells in the body. The metabolic defect in types A and B is insufficient activity of an enzyme called sphingomyelinase that initiates the biodegradation of sphingomyelin that arises from normal cell turnover. The term NP also includes 2 other variant forms called types C and D. Patients with these types have only moderate enlargement of their spleens and livers. They have brain involvement that can be extensive leading to inability to look up and down, difficulty in walking and swallowing, as well as progressive loss of vision and hearing. The disorder may appear early in life or its onset may be delayed into the teen years. Both types are characterized by an inability to mobilize cholesterol in the nerve cells in the brain where it accumulates and causes malfunction of these cells. The only difference between these two subtypes is that type D arises in people with a common ancestral background in Nova Scotia.

Is There Any Treatment?

There is currently no effective treatment for patients with type A. Bone marrow transplantation has been attempted in a few patients with type B, and encouraging results have been reported. Since type B resembles type 1 Gaucher's disease to a considerable degree, one might anticipate that enzyme replacement, and ultimately gene therapy, will eventually be helpful for these patients. Patients with types C and D are frequently placed on a low-cholesterol dietary regimen, but its clinical benefit is not convincing.

What Is the Prognosis?

Patients with type A die in infancy. Type B patients may live a comparatively long time, but many require supplemental oxygen because of lung involvement. The life expectancies of patients with types C and D are quite variable. Some patients die in childhood while others who appear to be less drastically affected live into adulthood.

What Research Is Being Done?

The gene that is altered in the majority of patients with type C (and D) was identified by investigators at NINDS. A second (different) gene that is mutated in a minority of patients with type C Niemann-Pick disease was discovered in 2000.

For More Information

For more information, contact:

Ara Parseghian Medical Research Foundation [For Niemann-Pick Type C Disease]
1760 East River Road
Suite 115
Tucson, AZ 85718
victory@parseghian.org
http://www.parseghian.org
Tel: 520-577-5106
Fax: 520-577-5212

National Niemann-Pick Disease Foundation, Inc.
P.O. Box 49
Ft. Atkinson, WI 53538
nnpdf@idcnet.com
http://www.nnpdf.org
Tel: 920-563-0930 / 877-CURE-NPC (287-3672)

National Tay-Sachs and Allied Diseases Association
2001 Beacon Street
Suite 204
Boston, MA 02135
NTSAD-boston@worldnet.att.net
http://www.ntsad.org
Tel: 617-277-4463 / 800-90-NTSAD (906-8723)
Fax: 617-277-0134

National Foundation for Jewish Genetic Diseases
250 Park Avenue
c/o Suite 1000
New York, NY 10177

http://www.nfjgd.org
Tel: 212-371-1030

More Guideline Sources

The guideline above on Niemann-Pick disease is only one example of the kind of material that you can find online and free of charge. The remainder of this chapter will direct you to other sources which either publish or can help you find additional guidelines on topics related to Niemann-Pick disease. Many of the guidelines listed below address topics that may be of particular relevance to your child's specific situation, while certain guidelines will apply to only some children with Niemann-Pick disease. Due to space limitations these sources are listed in a concise manner. Do not hesitate to consult the following sources by either using the Internet hyperlink provided, or, in cases where the contact information is provided, contacting the publisher or author directly.

Topic Pages: MEDLINEplus

For parents wishing to go beyond guidelines published by specific Institutes of the NIH, the National Library of Medicine has created a vast and parent-oriented healthcare information portal called MEDLINEplus. Within this Internet-based system are "health topic pages." You can think of a health topic page as a guide to patient guides. To access this system, log on to **http://www.nlm.nih.gov/medlineplus/healthtopics.html**. From there you can either search using the alphabetical index or browse by broad topic areas.

If you do not find topics of interest when browsing health topic pages, then you can choose to use the advanced search utility of MEDLINEplus at **http://www.nlm.nih.gov/medlineplus/advancedsearch.html**. This utility is similar to the NIH Search Utility, with the exception that it only includes material linked within the MEDLINEplus system (mostly parent-oriented information). It also has the disadvantage of generating unstructured results. We recommend, therefore, that you use this method only if you have a very targeted search.

The Combined Health Information Database (CHID)

CHID Online is a reference tool that maintains a database directory of thousands of journal articles and educational guidelines on Niemann-Pick disease and related conditions. One of the advantages of CHID over other sources is that it offers summaries that describe the guidelines available, including contact information and pricing. CHID's general Web site is **http://chid.nih.gov/**. To search this database, go to **http://chid.nih.gov/detail/detail.html**. In particular, you can use the advanced search options to look up pamphlets, reports, brochures, and information kits. The following was recently posted in this archive:

- **National Niemann Pick Disease Foundation**

    Source: Carrolltown, VA: National Niemann-Pick Disease Foundation, Inc. 1995. 6 p.

    Contact: Available from National Niemann-Pick Disease Foundation, Inc. 22201 Riverpoint Trail, Carrolltown, VA 23314-3917. (804) 357-6774. Price: Free.

    Summary: This brochure discusses Niemann-Pick disease. It talks about the signs and symptoms, how the disease is diagnosed, what treatment is available and how it is transmitted. It also gives background on the National Niemann-Pick Disease Foundation and the services it provides to families.

Healthfinder™

Healthfinder™ is an additional source sponsored by the U.S. Department of Health and Human Services which offers links to hundreds of other sites that contain healthcare information. This Web site is located at **http://www.healthfinder.gov**. Again, keyword searches can be used to find guidelines. The following was recently found in this database:

- **Niemann-Pick Disease**

    Summary: A general overview of Niemann-Pick disease that includes a description of the disorder, and treatment, prognosis and research information.

    Source: National Institute of Neurological Disorders and Stroke, National Institutes of Health

    http://www.healthfinder.gov/scripts/recordpass.asp?RecordType=0&RecordID=785

The NIH Search Utility

After browsing the references listed at the beginning of this chapter, you may want to explore the NIH Search Utility. This allows you to search for documents on over 100 selected Web sites that comprise the NIH-WEB-SPACE. Each of these servers is "crawled" and indexed on an ongoing basis. Your search will produce a list of various documents, all of which will relate in some way to Niemann-Pick disease. The drawbacks of this approach are that the information is not organized by theme and that the references are often a mix of information for professionals and parents. Nevertheless, a large number of the listed Web sites provide useful background information. We can only recommend this route, therefore, for relatively rare or specific disorders, or when using highly targeted searches. To use the NIH search utility, visit the following Web page: **http://search.nih.gov/index.html**.

Additional Web Sources

A number of Web sites that often link to government sites are available to the public. These can also point you in the direction of essential information. The following is a representative sample:

- AOL: **http://search.aol.com/cat.adp?id=168&layer=&from=subcats**
- drkoop.com®: **http://www.drkoop.com/conditions/ency/index.html**
- Family Village: **http://www.familyvillage.wisc.edu/specific.htm**
- Google: **http://directory.google.com/Top/Health/Conditions_and_Diseases/**
- Med Help International: **http://www.medhelp.org/HealthTopics/A.html**
- Open Directory Project: **http://dmoz.org/Health/Conditions_and_Diseases/**
- Yahoo.com: **http://dir.yahoo.com/Health/Diseases_and_Conditions/**
- WebMD®Health: **http://my.webmd.com/health_topics**

Vocabulary Builder

The material in this chapter may have contained a number of unfamiliar words. The following Vocabulary Builder introduces you to terms used in this chapter that have not been covered in the previous chapter:

Biodegradation: The series of processes by which living systems render chemicals less noxious to the environment. [EU]

Cholesterol: The principal sterol of all higher animals, distributed in body tissues, especially the brain and spinal cord, and in animal fats and oils. [NIH]

Enzyme: A protein molecule that catalyses chemical reactions of other substances without itself being destroyed or altered upon completion of the reactions. Enzymes are classified according to the recommendations of the Nomenclature Committee of the International Union of Biochemistry. Each enzyme is assigned a recommended name and an Enzyme Commission (EC) number. They are divided into six main groups; oxidoreductases, transferases, hydrolases, lyases, isomerases, and ligases. [EU]

Lipid: Any of a heterogeneous group of flats and fatlike substances characterized by being water-insoluble and being extractable by nonpolar (or fat) solvents such as alcohol, ether, chloroform, benzene, etc. All contain as a major constituent aliphatic hydrocarbons. The lipids, which are easily stored in the body, serve as a source of fuel, are an important constituent of cell structure, and serve other biological functions. Lipids may be considered to include fatty acids, neutral fats, waxes, and steroids. Compound lipids comprise the glycolipids, lipoproteins, and phospholipids. [EU]

Membrane: A thin layer of tissue which covers a surface, lines a cavity or divides a space or organ. [EU]

Progressive: Advancing; going forward; going from bad to worse; increasing in scope or severity. [EU]

Pulmonary: Pertaining to the lungs. [EU]

Transplantation: The grafting of tissues taken from the patient's own body or from another. [EU]

Chapter 2. Seeking Guidance

Overview

Some parents are comforted by the knowledge that a number of organizations dedicate their resources to helping people with Niemann-Pick disease. These associations can become invaluable sources of information and advice. Many associations offer parent support, financial assistance, and other important services. Furthermore, healthcare research has shown that support groups often help people to better cope with their conditions.[9] In addition to support groups, your child's physician can be a valuable source of guidance and support.

In this chapter, we direct you to resources that can help you find parent organizations and medical specialists. We begin by describing how to find associations and parent groups that can help you better understand and cope with your child's condition. The chapter ends with a discussion on how to find a doctor that is right for your child.

Associations and Niemann-Pick Disease

In addition to associations or groups that your child's doctor might recommend, we suggest that you consider the following list (if there is a fee for an association, you may want to check with your child's insurance provider to find out if the cost will be covered):

---

[9] Churches, synagogues, and other houses of worship might also have groups that can offer you the social support you need.

- **Ara Parseghian Medical Research Foundation**

    Address: Ara Parseghian Medical Research Foundation 1760 East River Road, Suite 115, Tucson, AZ 85718

    Telephone: (520) 577-5106 Toll-free: (800) 527-8005

    Fax: (520) 577-5212

    Email: victory@parseghien.org

    Web Site: http://www.parseghian.org

    Background: The Ara Parseghian Medical Research Foundation is an international not-for-profit voluntary organization dedicated to funding research projects to expedite a cure for Niemann-Pick Disease Type C (NP-C); promoting collaborative research efforts among the world's leading experts in cholesterol metabolism; and studying parallel pediatric neurodegenerative disorders. NP-C, a rare inherited disorder of childhood, is a degenerative disease that causes progressive deterioration of the nervous system due to an inability to properly break down cholesterol. Excessive amounts of cholesterol accumulate in the brain, liver, and spleen leading to a variety of symptoms and findings. These may include abnormal enlargement of the liver and spleen (hepatosplenomegaly); difficulty walking (ataxia) and positioning the arms and legs; slurred or slow speech; difficulties performing certain eye movements (vertical supranuclear gaze palsy); and additional symptoms. During mid-adolescence, progressive neurological problems usually lead to life-threatening complications. Established in 1994, the Foundation's purpose is to speed the search for a cure by funding research and promoting worldwide interaction among scientists, research institutes, and universities working on NP-C and related diseases involving the metabolism of cholesterol. Since its inception, the Foundation has raised more that $8 million and funds 20 research laboratories. A key element in the Foundation's focused research program is a Scientific Advisory Board including internationally recognized geneticists, molecular biologists, and pathologists who formulate the direction of Foundation-sponsored research and recommend grant proposals for funding. The Ara Parseghian Medical Research Foundation provides a variety of materials including informational packets, article reprints, brochures, and a regular newsletter entitled 'A Goal for Life.' The Foundation also has a web site on the Internet at http://www.parseghian.org.

- **Children's Liver Disease Foundation (UK)**

    Address: Children's Liver Disease Foundation (UK) AXA Equity and Law House, 35-37 Great Charles Street Queensway, Birmingham, B3 3JY, United Kingdom

Telephone: 0121 212 3839 Toll-free: (800) 527-8005

Fax: 0121 212 4300 E-

Web Site: http://www.childliverdisease.org

Background: The Children's Liver Disease Foundation (UK) is a voluntary not- for-profit organization in the United Kingdom that was established in 1980. The Foundation is committed to providing emotional support to children, adolescents, and families affected by liver disease; promoting research into the causes of pediatric liver disease; creating a greater awareness of such disorders and conditions in the health care communities and the public; and promoting the development of means of early diagnosis and cure. The Children's Liver Disease Foundation is also dedicated to providing understandable information on pediatric liver disease through general informational brochures including 'A Guide to the Liver' and 'Signs and Symptoms of Liver Disease' as well as a leaflet series on specific pediatric liver diseases and conditions, such as Alagille syndrome; neonatal hepatitis; hepatitis A, B, C, and E; biliary atresia; and others. The Foundation's web site on the Internet discusses the organization's mission, goals, and services; enables interested individuals, family members, and health care professionals to make specific inquiries; and provides access to the Foundation's publication series.

Relevant area(s) of interest: Niemann Pick Disease

- **March of Dimes Birth Defects Foundation**

    Address: March of Dimes Birth Defects Foundation 1275 Mamaroneck Avenue, White Plains, NY 10605

    Telephone: (914) 428-7100 Toll-free: (888) 663-4637

    Fax: (914) 997-4763

    Email: resourcecenter@modimes.org

    Web Site: http://www.modimes.org

    Background: The March of Dimes Birth Defects Foundation is a national not-for- profit organization that was established in 1938. The mission of the Foundation is to improve the health of babies by preventing birth defects and infant mortality. Through the Campaign for Healthier Babies, the March of Dimes funds programs of research, community services, education, and advocacy. Educational programs that seek to prevent birth defects are important to the Foundation and to that end it produces a wide variety of printed informational materials and videos. The March of Dimes public health educational materials provide information encouraging health- enhancing behaviors that lead to a healthy pregnancy and a healthy baby.

Relevant area(s) of interest: Leigh's Disease, Menkes Disease, Mucopolysaccharidoses, Niemann Pick Disease, Refsum Disease, Sandhoff Disease

- **National Foundation for Jewish Genetic Diseases**

  Address: National Foundation for Jewish Genetic Diseases 250 Park Avenue, Suite 1000, New York, NY 10017

  Telephone: (212) 371-1030 Toll-free: (888) 663-4637

  Fax: (212) 319-5808

  Background: The National Foundation for Jewish Genetic Diseases is a not-for- profit voluntary health and research organization devoted to supporting medical research and informing the public and medical communities about the seven most common Jewish genetic diseases. These diseases include Gaucher Disease, Dystonia, Familial Dysautonomia, Tay-Sach's Disease, Bloom Syndrome, Niemann-Pick Disease, and Mucolipidosis IV. The National Foundation for Jewish Genetic Diseases aims to advance progress toward the cure and/or prevention of these disorders. The major efforts of the Foundation are directed to help physicians and researchers understand the nature of these rare genetic diseases so that newer and better means of diagnosis, management, treatment, and prevention can be developed. Informational fact sheets on each of these diseases are produced by the Foundation and describe the specific nature of the genetic defect, diagnostic tests, and available disease management and treatments. The National Foundation for Jewish Genetic Diseases also supports research and training programs through endowed scholarship programs and direct funding to academic and medical research centers.

  Relevant area(s) of interest: Niemann Pick Disease

- **National Lipid Diseases Foundation**

  Address: National Lipid Diseases Foundation 1201 Corbin Street, Elizabeth, NJ 07201

  Telephone: (908) 527-8000 Toll-free: (800) 527-8005

  Fax: (908) 527-8004

  Background: Established in 1965, the National Lipid Diseases Foundation is a voluntary not-for-profit organization dedicated to raising research funds for lipid storage diseases. Lipid storage diseases are a group of rare inherited metabolic disorders characterized by an abnormal accumulation of lipids (fatty or fatty-like substances) in different tissues of the body. Symptoms may vary greatly and depend on the affected organ system(s). The Foundation's funds currently go to Columbia Presbyterian Hospital to purchase research equipment and to Massachusetts General Hospital to support clinical research on Gaucher's Disease. The National Lipid Diseases Foundation provides referrals to those who are interested in receiving genetic counseling and/or educational materials concerning lipid storage diseases.

Relevant area(s) of interest: Niemann Pick Disease, Sandhoff Disease

- **National Niemann-Pick Disease Foundation, Inc**

    Address: National Niemann-Pick Disease Foundation, Inc. 3734 East Olive Avenue, Gilbert, AZ 85234-3117

    Telephone: (602) 497-6638 Toll-free: (888) 663-4637

    Fax: (602) 497-6346

    Email: stevekenyon@netwrx.net

    Web Site: http://www.nnpdf.org/

    Background: The National Niemann-Pick Disease Foundation, Inc. is an international voluntary not-for-profit organization made up of parents, medical professionals, friends, relatives, and others who are committed to finding a cure for Niemann-Pick Disease (NPD). Niemann-Pick is a group of rare inherited diseases in which excessive amounts of a fatty substance called sphingomyelin and/or cholesterol accumulate in many organs of the body. Established in 1984, the National Niemann-Pick Disease Foundation is dedicated to promoting medical research into the cause and cure of Niemann- Pick Disease; providing medical and educational information to assist in the correct diagnosis and referral of children with Niemann-Pick Disease; and providing support to families of affected children. The Foundation is also committed to facilitating genetic counseling for parents who are known carriers of Niemann-Pick Disease; encouraging the sharing of research information among scientists; and supporting legislation that is beneficial to affected individuals and family members. The National Niemann-Pick Disease Foundation also conducts a national conference that gives families the opportunity to network with one another and meet with medical professionals and researchers. The Foundation provides a variety of educational and support materials through its database, directory, reports, regular newsletter, and brochures.

    Relevant area(s) of interest: Niemann Pick Disease

- **National Tay-Sachs and Allied Diseases Association, Inc**

    Address: National Tay-Sachs and Allied Diseases Association, Inc. 2001 Beacon Street, Suite 204, Brookline, MA 02135

    Telephone: (617) 277-4463 Toll-free: (800) 906-8723

    Fax: (617) 277-0134

    Email: NTSAD- Boston@worldnet.att.net

    Web Site: http://www.NTSAD.org

    Background: The National Tay-Sachs and Allied Diseases Association, Inc. (NTSAD) is a voluntary not-for-profit health organization dedicated to the prevention and eradication of Tay-Sachs and 40 related genetic disorders. Established in 1956, the Association has expanded to encompass active chapters in major metropolitan areas, a Scientific Advisory Committee, and a Parent Peer Support Group that extends worldwide. Through the guidance and expertise of its Scientific Advisory Committee, the Association promotes Tay-Sachs carrier screening, sponsors a Tay-Sachs Laboratory Quality Control Program, and publishes a current listing of participating labs. It approves candidates for research fellowships and maintains a repository of specialized knowledge for affected individuals, family members, health care professionals, and others who seek a greater understanding of lysosomal storage diseases. The Association also conducts an annual conference and provides support, referral, and advocacy services from its national office and affiliate chapters. In addition, the National Tay-Sachs and Allied Diseases Association offers a variety of educational and support materials. These materials include a directory of families, a directory of Tay-Sachs Test Centers, regular newsletters, fact sheets, brochures, videos, and a child care manual. The Association also provides a lending library and a traveling educational display.

    Relevant area(s) of interest: Mucopolysaccharidoses, Niemann Pick Disease, Sandhoff Disease

- **Research Trust for Metabolic Diseases in Children**

    Address: Research Trust for Metabolic Diseases in Children The Quadrangle, Crewe Hall, Weston Road, Crewe, Cheshire, CW1 6UR, United Kingdom

    Telephone: 1270 250221

    Fax: 1270 250244

    Web Site: http://www.RTMDC.org.uk

Background: The Research Trust for Metabolic Diseases in Children (RTMDC) is an international voluntary health agency located in the United Kingdom. Established in 1981, the Trust is dedicated to furthering medical research into the nature of metabolic diseases in children; encouraging the ongoing investigations of the prenatal diagnosis of these diseases; providing information, counseling, and financial support to caregivers; and providing information to health care professionals. In addition, the organization is dedicated to assisting in the care of affected children in hospitals, homes, or institutions and educating the public about metabolic diseases. The Research Trust for Metabolic Diseases networks parents of affected children for mutual benefit and support. The Trust also provides a regular newsletter, brochures, videos, and other educational materials.

Relevant area(s) of interest: Niemann Pick Disease, Refsum Disease

- **Vaincre Les Maladies Lysosomales**

  Address: Vaincre Les Maladies Lysosomales 9 Place du 19 Mars 1962,, Evry Cedex, 91035, France

  Telephone: (331) 609-1750

  Fax: 3(316) 936-9350

  Email: VML@provnet.fr

  Web Site: http://www.provnet.fr/VML/

  Background: Vaincre Les Maladies Lysosomales is a voluntary not-for-profit organization in France dedicated to providing information and support to individuals with lysosomal disorders and their families; improving the quality of life of affected individuals; and promoting and supporting research for these disorders (e.g., Pompe Disease, the Lipidoses, Mucolipidoses, Mucopolysaccharidoses, and Glycoproteinoses). Established in 1990, Vaincre Les Maladies Lysosomales provides referrals to appropriate support groups; promotes public awareness campaigns; and offers informational conferences and weekend retreats for affected individuals, families, and health care professionals. Vaincre Les Maladies Lysosomales also offers a variety of educational materials to affected individuals, family members, and health care professionals including regular newsletters, brochures, books, and videos.

  Relevant area(s) of interest: Mucopolysaccharidoses, Niemann Pick Disease, Sandhoff Disease

Finding More Associations

There are a number of directories that list additional medical associations that you may find useful. While not all of these directories will provide different information than what is listed above, by consulting all of them, you will have nearly exhausted all sources for parent associations.

The National Health Information Center (NHIC)

The National Health Information Center (NHIC) offers a free referral service to help people find organizations that provide information about Niemann-Pick disease. For more information, see the NHIC's Web site at **http://www.health.gov/NHIC/** or contact an information specialist by calling 1-800-336-4797.

DIRLINE

A comprehensive source of information on associations is the DIRLINE database maintained by the National Library of Medicine. The database comprises some 10,000 records of organizations, research centers, and government institutes and associations which primarily focus on health and biomedicine. DIRLINE is available via the Internet at the following Web site: **http://dirline.nlm.nih.gov**. Simply type in "Niemann-Pick disease" (or a synonym) or the name of a topic, and the site will list information contained in the database on all relevant organizations.

The Combined Health Information Database

Another comprehensive source of information on healthcare associations is the Combined Health Information Database. Using the "Detailed Search" option, you will need to limit your search to "Organizations" and "Niemann-Pick disease". Type the following hyperlink into your Web browser: **http://chid.nih.gov/detail/detail.html**. To find associations, use the drop boxes at the bottom of the search page where "You may refine your search by." For publication date, select "All Years." Then, select your preferred language and the format option "Organization Resource Sheet." By making these selections and typing in "Niemann-Pick disease" (or synonyms) into the "For these words:" box, you will only receive results on organizations dealing with Niemann-Pick disease. You should check back periodically with this database since it is updated every 3 months.

The National Organization for Rare Disorders, Inc.

The National Organization for Rare Disorders, Inc. has prepared a Web site that provides, at no charge, lists of associations organized by specific medical conditions. You can access this database at the following Web site: **http://www.rarediseases.org/cgi-bin/nord/searchpage**. Select the option called "Organizational Database (ODB)" and type "Niemann-Pick disease" (or a synonym) in the search box.

Online Support Groups

In addition to support groups, commercial Internet service providers offer forums and chat rooms to discuss different illnesses and conditions. WebMD®, for example, offers such a service at their Web site: **http://boards.webmd.com/roundtable**. These online communities can help you connect with a network of people whose concerns are similar to yours. Online support groups are places where people can talk informally. If you read about a novel approach, consult with your child's doctor or other healthcare providers, as the treatments or discoveries you hear about may not be scientifically proven to be safe and effective.

Finding Doctors

All parents must go through the process of selecting a physician for their children with Niemann-Pick disease. While this process will vary, the Agency for Healthcare Research and Quality makes a number of suggestions, including the following:[10]

- If your child is in a managed care plan, check the plan's list of doctors first.
- Ask doctors or other health professionals who work with doctors, such as hospital nurses, for referrals.
- Call a hospital's doctor referral service, but keep in mind that these services usually refer you to doctors on staff at that particular hospital. The services do not have information on the quality of care that these doctors provide.
- Some local medical societies offer lists of member doctors. Again, these lists do not have information on the quality of care that these doctors provide.

---

[10] This section is adapted from the AHRQ: www.ahrq.gov/consumer/qntascii/qntdr.htm.

Additional steps you can take to locate doctors include the following:
- Check with the associations listed earlier in this chapter.
- Information on doctors in some states is available on the Internet at **http://www.docboard.org**. This Web site is run by "Administrators in Medicine," a group of state medical board directors.
- The American Board of Medical Specialties can tell you if your child's doctor is board certified. "Certified" means that the doctor has completed a training program in a specialty and has passed an exam, or "board," to assess his or her knowledge, skills, and experience to provide quality patient care in that specialty. Primary care doctors may also be certified as specialists. The AMBS Web site is located at **http://www.abms.org/newsearch.asp**.[11] You can also contact the ABMS by phone at 1-866-ASK-ABMS.
- You can call the American Medical Association (AMA) at 800-665-2882 for information on training, specialties, and board certification for many licensed doctors in the United States. This information also can be found in "Physician Select" at the AMA's Web site: **http://www.ama-assn.org/aps/amahg.htm**.

If the previous sources did not meet your needs, you may want to log on to the Web site of the National Organization for Rare Disorders (NORD) at **http://www.rarediseases.org/**. NORD maintains a database of doctors with expertise in various rare medical conditions. The Metabolic Information Network (MIN), 800-945-2188, also maintains a database of physicians with expertise in various metabolic diseases.

Finding a Neurologist

The American Academy of Neurology allows you to search for member neurologists by name or location. To use this service, go to **http://www.aan.com/**, select "Find a Neurologist" from the toolbar. Enter your search criteria, and click "Search." To find out more information on a particular neurologist, click on the physician's name.

If the previous sources did not meet your needs, you may want to log on to the Web site of the National Organization for Rare Disorders (NORD) at **http://www.rarediseases.org/**. NORD maintains a database of doctors with expertise in various rare diseases. The Metabolic Information Network

---

[11] While board certification is a good measure of a doctor's knowledge, it is possible to receive quality care from doctors who are not board certified.

(MIN), 800-945-2188, also maintains a database of physicians with expertise in various metabolic diseases.

Selecting Your Doctor[2]

When you have compiled a list of prospective doctors, call each of their offices. First, ask if the doctor accepts your child's health insurance plan and if he or she is taking new patients. If the doctor is not covered by your child's plan, ask yourself if you are prepared to pay the extra costs. The next step is to schedule a visit with your first choice. During the first visit you will have the opportunity to evaluate your child's doctor and to find out if your child feels comfortable with him or her.

Working with Your Child's Doctor[13]

Research has shown that parents who have good relationships with their children's doctors tend to be more satisfied with their children's care. Here are some tips to help you and your child's doctor become partners:

- You know important things about your child's symptoms and health history. Tell the doctor what you think he or she needs to know.
- Always bring any medications your child is currently taking with you to the appointment, or you can bring a list of your child's medications including dosage and frequency information. Talk about any allergies or reactions your child has had to medications.
- Tell your doctor about any natural or alternative medicines your child is taking.
- Bring other medical information, such as x-ray films, test results, and medical records.
- Ask questions. If you don't, the doctor will assume that you understood everything that was said.
- Write down your questions before the doctor's visit. List the most important ones first to make sure that they are addressed.
- Ask the doctor to draw pictures if you think that this will help you and your child understand.

---

[12] This section has been adapted from the AHRQ: www.ahrq.gov/consumer/qntascii/qntdr.htm.
[13] This section has been adapted from the AHRQ: www.ahrq.gov/consumer/qntascii/qntdr.htm.

- Take notes. Some doctors do not mind if you bring a tape recorder to help you remember things, but always ask first.
- Take information home. Ask for written instructions. Your child's doctor may also have brochures and audio and videotapes on Niemann-Pick disease.

By following these steps, you will enhance the relationship you and your child have with the physician.

Broader Health-Related Resources

In addition to the references above, the NIH has set up guidance Web sites that can help parents find healthcare professionals. These include:[14]

- Caregivers:
  http://www.nlm.nih.gov/medlineplus/caregivers.html
- Choosing a Doctor or Healthcare Service:
  http://www.nlm.nih.gov/medlineplus/choosingadoctororhealthcareservice.html
- Hospitals and Health Facilities:
  http://www.nlm.nih.gov/medlineplus/healthfacilities.html

Vocabulary Builder

The following vocabulary builder provides definitions of words used in this chapter that have not been defined in previous chapters:

Adolescence: The period of life beginning with the appearance of secondary sex characteristics and terminating with the cessation of somatic growth. The years usually referred to as adolescence lie between 13 and 18 years of age. [NIH]

Ataxia: Failure of muscular coordination; irregularity of muscular action. [EU]

Biliary: Pertaining to the bile, to the bile ducts, or to the gallbladder. [EU]

Dystonia: Disordered tonicity of muscle. [EU]

Hepatitis: Inflammation of the liver. [EU]

---

[14] You can access this information at:
http://www.nlm.nih.gov/medlineplus/healthsystem.html.

Molecular: Of, pertaining to, or composed of molecules : a very small mass of matter. [EU]

Neonatal: Pertaining to the first four weeks after birth. [EU]

Neurology: A medical specialty concerned with the study of the structures, functions, and diseases of the nervous system. [NIH]

Prenatal: Existing or occurring before birth, with reference to the fetus. [EU]

CHAPTER 3. CLINICAL TRIALS AND NIEMANN-PICK DISEASE

Overview

Very few medical conditions have a single treatment. The basic treatment guidelines that your child's physician has discussed with you, or those that you have found using the techniques discussed in Chapter 1, may provide you with all that you will require. For some patients, current treatments can be enhanced with new or innovative techniques currently under investigation. In this chapter, we will describe how clinical trials work and show you how to keep informed of trials concerning Niemann-Pick disease.

What Is a Clinical Trial?[15]

Clinical trials involve the participation of people in medical research. Most medical research begins with studies in test tubes and on animals. Treatments that show promise in these early studies may then be tried with people. The only sure way to find out whether a new treatment is safe, effective, and better than other treatments for Niemann-Pick disease is to try it on patients in a clinical trial.

---

[15] The discussion in this chapter has been adapted from the NIH and the NEI: www.nei.nih.gov/netrials/ctivr.htm.

What Kinds of Clinical Trials Are There?

Clinical trials are carried out in three phases:
- **Phase I.** Researchers first conduct Phase I trials with small numbers of patients and healthy volunteers. If the new treatment is a medication, researchers also try to determine how much of it can be given safely.
- **Phase II.** Researchers conduct Phase II trials in small numbers of patients to find out the effect of a new treatment on Niemann-Pick disease.
- **Phase III.** Finally, researchers conduct Phase III trials to find out how new treatments for Niemann-Pick disease compare with standard treatments already being used. Phase III trials also help to determine if new treatments have any side effects. These trials--which may involve hundreds, perhaps thousands, of people--can also compare new treatments with no treatment.

How Is a Clinical Trial Conducted?

Various organizations support clinical trials at medical centers, hospitals, universities, and doctors' offices across the United States. The "principal investigator" is the researcher in charge of the study at each facility participating in the clinical trial. Most clinical trial researchers are medical doctors, academic researchers, and specialists. The "clinic coordinator" knows all about how the study works and makes all the arrangements for your child's visits.

All doctors and researchers who take part in the study on Niemann-Pick disease carefully follow a detailed treatment plan called a protocol. This plan fully explains how the doctors will treat your child in the study. The "protocol" ensures that all patients are treated in the same way, no matter where they receive care.

Clinical trials are controlled. This means that researchers compare the effects of the new treatment with those of the standard treatment. In some cases, when no standard treatment exists, the new treatment is compared with no treatment. Patients who receive the new treatment are in the treatment group. Patients who receive a standard treatment or no treatment are in the "control" group. In some clinical trials, patients in the treatment group get a new medication while those in the control group get a placebo. A placebo is a harmless substance, a "dummy" pill, that has no effect on Niemann-Pick disease. In other clinical trials, where a new surgery or device (not a medicine) is being tested, patients in the control group may receive a "sham treatment." This treatment, like a placebo, has no effect on Niemann-Pick disease and will not harm your child.

Researchers assign patients "randomly" to the treatment or control group. This is like flipping a coin to decide which patients are in each group. If you choose to have your child participate in a clinical trial, you will not know which group he or she will be appointed to. The chance of any patient getting the new treatment is about 50 percent. You cannot request that your child receive the new treatment instead of the placebo or "sham" treatment. Often, you will not know until the study is over whether your child has been in the treatment group or the control group. This is called a "masked" study. In some trials, neither doctors nor patients know who is getting which treatment. This is called a "double masked" study. These types of trials help to ensure that the perceptions of the participants or doctors will not affect the study results.

Natural History Studies

Unlike clinical trials in which patient volunteers may receive new treatments, natural history studies provide important information to researchers on how Niemann-Pick disease develops over time. A natural history study follows patient volunteers to see how factors such as age, sex, race, or family history might make some people more or less at risk for Niemann-Pick disease. A natural history study may also tell researchers if diet, lifestyle, or occupation affects how a medical condition develops and progresses. Results from these studies provide information that helps answer questions such as: How fast will a medical condition usually progress? How bad will the condition become? Will treatment be needed?

What Is Expected of Your Child in a Clinical Trial?

Not everyone can take part in a clinical trial for a specific medical condition. Each study enrolls patients with certain features or eligibility criteria. These criteria may include the type and stage of the condition, as well as, the age and previous treatment history of the patient. You or your child's doctor can contact the sponsoring organization to find out more about specific clinical trials and their eligibility criteria. If you would like your child to participate in a clinical trial, your child's doctor must contact one of the trial's investigators and provide details about his or her diagnosis and medical history.

When participating in a clinical trial, your child may be required to have a number of medical tests. Your child may also need to take medications and/or undergo surgery. Depending upon the treatment and the examination procedure, your child may be required to receive inpatient hospital care. He or she may have to return to the medical facility for follow-up examinations. These exams help find out how well the treatment is working. Follow-up studies can take months or years. However, the success of the clinical trial often depends on learning what happens to patients over a long period of time. Only patients who continue to return for follow-up examinations can provide this important long-term information.

Recent Trials on Niemann-Pick Disease

The National Institutes of Health and other organizations sponsor trials on various medical conditions. Because funding for research goes to the medical areas that show promising research opportunities, it is not possible for the NIH or others to sponsor clinical trials for every medical condition at all times. The following lists recent trials dedicated to Niemann-Pick disease.[16] If the trial listed by the NIH is still recruiting, your child may be eligible. If it is no longer recruiting or has been completed, then you can contact the sponsors to learn more about the study and, if published, the results. Further information on the trial is available at the Web site indicated. Please note that some trials may no longer be recruiting patients or are otherwise closed. Before contacting sponsors of a clinical trial, consult with your child's physician who can help you determine if your child might benefit from participation.

- **PET Scan of Brain Metabolism in Relation to Age and Disease**

    Condition(s): Alzheimer's Disease; Brain Neoplasm; Niemann Pick Disease

    Study Status: This study is completed.

    Sponsor(s): National Institute of Neurological Disorders and Stroke (NINDS)

    Purpose - Excerpt: The main source of energy for the brain comes from a combination of oxygen and glucose (sugar). For brain cells to function normally they must receive a constant supply of these nutrients. As areas of the brain become more active blood flow into and out of these areas increase. In addition to oxygen and glucose, the brain uses chemical compounds known as phospholipids. These phosopholipids make up the covering of nerve cells that assist in the transfer of information from cell

---

[16] These are listed at www.ClinicalTrials.gov.

to cell. Without phospholipids brain cell activity may become abnormal and cause problems in the nervous system. Certain diseases like Alzheimer's disease and brain tumors can affect blood flow to the brain and change the way the brain metabolizes phopholipids. In addition to diseases, changes in the brain occur with normal healthy aging. This study is designed to use PET scan to measure changes in blood flow and changes in phopholipid metabolism. Using this technique, researchers can improve their understanding of how certain diseases change the shape and function of the brain.

Study Type: Observational

Contact(s): Maryland; National Institute of Neurological Disorders and Stroke (NINDS), 9000 Rockville Pike Bethesda, Maryland, 20892, United States

Web Site:
http://clinicaltrials.gov/ct/gui/show/NCT00001972;jsessionid=333877051316D342E552434999262963

Benefits and Risks[17]

What Are the Benefits of Participating in a Clinical Trial?

If you are considering a clinical trial, it is important to realize that your child's participation can bring many benefits:

- A new treatment could be more effective than the current treatment for Niemann-Pick disease. Although only half of the participants in a clinical trial receive the experimental treatment, if the new treatment is proved to be more effective and safer than the current treatment, then those patients who did not receive the new treatment during the clinical trial may be among the first to benefit from it when the study is over.

- If the treatment is effective, then it may improve your child's health.

- Clinical trial patients receive the highest quality of medical care. Experts watch them closely during the study and may continue to follow them after the study is over.

- People who take part in trials contribute to scientific discoveries that may help others with Niemann-Pick disease. In cases where certain medical

---

[17] This section has been adapted from ClinicalTrials.gov, a service of the National Institutes of Health:
http://www.clinicaltrials.gov/ct/gui/c/a1r/info/whatis?JServSessionIdzone_ct=9jmun6f291.

conditions run in families, your child's participation may lead to better care or prevention for you and other family members.

The Informed Consent

Once you agree to have your child take part in a clinical trial, you will be asked to sign an "informed consent." This document explains a clinical trial's risks and benefits, the researcher's expectations of you and your child, and your child's rights as a patient.

What Are the Risks?

Clinical trials may involve risks as well as benefits. Whether or not a new treatment will work cannot be known ahead of time. There is always a chance that a new treatment may not work better than a standard treatment. There is also the possibility that it may be harmful. The treatment your child receives may cause side effects that are serious enough to require medical attention.

How Is Your Child's Safety Protected?

Clinical trials can raise fears of the unknown. Understanding the safeguards that protect your child can ease some of these fears. Before a clinical trial begins, researchers must get approval from their hospital's Institutional Review Board (IRB), an advisory group that makes sure a clinical trial is designed to protect your child's safety. During a clinical trial, doctors will closely watch your child to see if the treatment is working and if he or she is experiencing any side effects. All the results are carefully recorded and reviewed. In many cases, experts from the Data and Safety Monitoring Committee carefully monitor each clinical trial and can recommend that a study be stopped at any time. Your child will only be asked to participate in a clinical trial as a volunteer with your informed consent.

What Are Your Child's Rights in a Clinical Trial?

If your child is eligible for a clinical trial, you will be given information to help you decide whether or not you want him or her to participate. You and your child have the right to:

- Information on all known risks and benefits of the treatments in the study.
- Know how the researchers plan to carry out the study, for how long, and where.
- Know what is expected of your child.
- Know any costs involved for you or your child's insurance provider.
- Know before any of your child's medical or personal information is shared with other researchers involved in the clinical trial.
- Talk openly with doctors and ask any questions.

After your child joins a clinical trial, you and your child have the right to:

- Leave the study at any time. Participation is strictly voluntary.
- Receive any new information about the new treatment.
- Continue to ask questions and get answers.
- Maintain your child's privacy. Your child's name will not appear in any reports based on the study.
- Know whether your child participated in the treatment group or the control group (once the study has been completed).

What about Costs?

In some clinical trials, the research facility pays for treatment costs and other associated expenses. You or your child's insurance provider may have to pay for costs that are considered standard care. These things may include inpatient hospital care, laboratory and other tests, and medical procedures. You also may need to pay for travel between your home and the clinic. You should find out about costs before committing your child to participation in the trial. If your child has health insurance, find out exactly what it will cover. If your child does not have health insurance, or if your child's insurance policy will not cover care, talk to the clinic staff about other options for covering the costs.

What Questions Should You Ask before Your Child Participates in a Clinical Trial?

Questions you should ask when deciding whether or not to enroll your child in a clinical trial include the following:

- What is the purpose of the clinical trial?
- What are the standard treatments for Niemann-Pick disease? Why do researchers think the new treatment may be better? What is likely to happen to my child with or without the new treatment?
- What tests and treatments will my child need? Will my child need surgery? Medication? Hospitalization?
- How long will the treatment last? How often will my child have to come back for follow-up exams?
- What are the treatment's possible benefits to my child's condition? What are the short- and long-term risks? What are the possible side effects?
- Will the treatment be uncomfortable? Will it make my child sick? If so, for how long?
- How will my child's health be monitored?
- Where will my child need to go for the clinical trial?
- How much will it cost to participate in the study? What costs are covered by the study? How much will my child's health insurance cover?
- Who will be in charge of my child's care?
- Will taking part in the study affect my child's daily life?
- How does my child feel about taking part in a clinical trial? Will other family members benefit from my child's contributions to new medical knowledge?

Keeping Current on Clinical Trials

Various government agencies maintain databases on trials. The U.S. National Institutes of Health, through the National Library of Medicine, has developed ClinicalTrials.gov to provide the public and physicians with current information about clinical research across the broadest number of medical conditions.

The site was launched in February 2000 and currently contains approximately 5,700 clinical studies in over 59,000 locations worldwide, with most studies being conducted in the United States. ClinicalTrials.gov receives about 2 million hits per month and hosts approximately 5,400 visitors daily. To access this database, simply go to their Web site (**www.clinicaltrials.gov**) and search by "Niemann-Pick disease" (or synonyms).

While ClinicalTrials.gov is the most comprehensive listing of NIH-supported clinical trials available, not all trials are in the database. The database is updated regularly, so clinical trials are continually being added. The following is a list of specialty databases affiliated with the National Institutes of Health that offer additional information on trials:

- For clinical studies at the Warren Grant Magnuson Clinical Center located in Bethesda, Maryland, visit their Web site:
  http://clinicalstudies.info.nih.gov/

- For clinical studies conducted at the Bayview Campus in Baltimore, Maryland, visit their Web site:
  http://www.jhbmc.jhu.edu/studies/index.html

- For trials on neurological disorders and stroke, visit and search the Web site sponsored by the National Institute of Neurological Disorders and Stroke of the NIH:
  http://www.ninds.nih.gov/funding/funding_opportunities.htm#Clinical_Trials

General References

The following references describe clinical trials and experimental medical research. They have been selected to ensure that they are likely to be available from your local or online bookseller or university medical library. These references are usually written for healthcare professionals, so you may consider consulting with a librarian or bookseller who might recommend a particular reference. The following includes some of the most readily available references (sorted alphabetically by title; hyperlinks provide rankings, information and reviews at Amazon.com):

- **A Guide to Patient Recruitment : Today's Best Practices & Proven Strategies** by Diana L. Anderson; Paperback - 350 pages (2001), CenterWatch, Inc.; ISBN: 1930624115;
  http://www.amazon.com/exec/obidos/ASIN/1930624115/icongroupinterna

- **A Step-By-Step Guide to Clinical Trials** by Marilyn Mulay, R.N., M.S., OCN; Spiral-bound - 143 pages Spiral edition (2001), Jones & Bartlett Pub; ISBN: 0763715697;
  http://www.amazon.com/exec/obidos/ASIN/0763715697/icongroupinterna

- **The CenterWatch Directory of Drugs in Clinical Trials** by CenterWatch; Paperback - 656 pages (2000), CenterWatch, Inc.; ISBN: 0967302935; http://www.amazon.com/exec/obidos/ASIN/0967302935/icongroupinterna
- **The Complete Guide to Informed Consent in Clinical Trials** by Terry Hartnett (Editor); Paperback - 164 pages (2000), PharmSource Information Services, Inc.; ISBN: 0970153309; http://www.amazon.com/exec/obidos/ASIN/0970153309/icongroupinterna
- **Dictionary for Clinical Trials** by Simon Day; Paperback - 228 pages (1999), John Wiley & Sons; ISBN: 0471985961; http://www.amazon.com/exec/obidos/ASIN/0471985961/icongroupinterna
- **Extending Medicare Reimbursement in Clinical Trials** by Institute of Medicine Staff (Editor), et al; Paperback 1st edition (2000), National Academy Press; ISBN: 0309068886; http://www.amazon.com/exec/obidos/ASIN/0309068886/icongroupinterna
- **Handbook of Clinical Trials** by Marcus Flather (Editor); Paperback (2001), Remedica Pub Ltd; ISBN: 1901346293; http://www.amazon.com/exec/obidos/ASIN/1901346293/icongroupinterna

Vocabulary Builder

The following vocabulary builder gives definitions of words used in this chapter that have not been defined in previous chapters:

Glucose: D-glucose, a monosaccharide (hexose), $C_6H_{12}O_6$, also known as dextrose (q.v.), found in certain foodstuffs, especially fruits, and in the normal blood of all animals. It is the end product of carbohydrate metabolism and is the chief source of energy for living organisms, its utilization being controlled by insulin. Excess glucose is converted to glycogen and stored in the liver and muscles for use as needed and, beyond that, is converted to fat and stored as adipose tissue. Glucose appears in the urine in diabetes mellitus. [EU]

PART II: ADDITIONAL RESOURCES AND ADVANCED MATERIAL

ABOUT PART II

In Part II, we introduce you to additional resources and advanced research on Niemann-Pick disease. All too often, parents who conduct their own research are overwhelmed by the difficulty in finding and organizing information. The purpose of the following chapters is to provide you an organized and structured format to help you find additional information resources on Niemann-Pick disease. In Part II, as in Part I, our objective is not to interpret the latest advances on Niemann-Pick disease or render an opinion. Rather, our goal is to give you access to original research and to increase your awareness of sources you may not have already considered. In this way, you will come across the advanced materials often referred to in pamphlets, books, or other general works. Once again, some of this material is technical in nature, so consultation with a professional familiar with Niemann-Pick disease is suggested.

CHAPTER 4. STUDIES ON NIEMANN-PICK DISEASE

Overview

Every year, academic studies are published on Niemann-Pick disease or related conditions. Broadly speaking, there are two types of studies. The first are peer reviewed. Generally, the content of these studies has been reviewed by scientists or physicians. Peer-reviewed studies are typically published in scientific journals and are usually available at medical libraries. The second type of studies is non-peer reviewed. These works include summary articles that do not use or report scientific results. These often appear in the popular press, newsletters, or similar periodicals.

In this chapter, we will show you how to locate peer-reviewed references and studies on Niemann-Pick disease. We will begin by discussing research that has been summarized and is free to view by the public via the Internet. We then show you how to generate a bibliography on Niemann-Pick disease and teach you how to keep current on new studies as they are published or undertaken by the scientific community.

Federally-Funded Research on Niemann-Pick Disease

The U.S. Government supports a variety of research studies relating to Niemann-Pick disease and associated conditions. These studies are tracked by the Office of Extramural Research at the National Institutes of Health.[18]

---

[18] Healthcare projects are funded by the National Institutes of Health (NIH), Substance Abuse and Mental Health Services (SAMHSA), Health Resources and Services Administration (HRSA), Food and Drug Administration (FDA), Centers for Disease Control and Prevention (CDCP), Agency for Healthcare Research and Quality (AHRQ), and Office of Assistant Secretary of Health (OASH).

CRISP (Computerized Retrieval of Information on Scientific Projects) is a searchable database of federally-funded biomedical research projects conducted at universities, hospitals, and other institutions. Visit the CRISP Web site at **http://commons.cit.nih.gov/crisp3/CRISP.Generate_Ticket**. You can perform targeted searches by various criteria including geography, date, as well as topics related to Niemann-Pick disease and related conditions.

For most of the studies, the agencies reporting into CRISP provide summaries or abstracts. As opposed to clinical trial research using patients, many federally-funded studies use animals or simulated models to explore Niemann-Pick disease and related conditions. In some cases, therefore, it may be difficult to understand how some basic or fundamental research could eventually translate into medical practice. The following sample is typical of the type of information found when searching the CRISP database for Niemann-Pick disease:

- **Project Title: Analysis of Niemann-Pick C Protein (NPCI) Function**

    Principal Investigator & Institution: Berger, Adam C.; Biochemistry; Emory University 1380 S Oxford Rd Atlanta, Ga 30322

    Timing: Fiscal Year 2002; Project Start 1-DEC-2002

    Summary: (provided by applicant): The broad, long-term objective of this proposal is to utilize the genetically tractable model organism, S. cerevisiae, to study the cellular function of the Niemann-Pick disease type C (NP-C) protein, NPC1. NP-C is a fatal neurodegenerative disorder with a prevalence of 1 in 150,000 live births. Biochemically, NP-C is a lipid storage disorder marked by the lysosomal accumulation of unesterified cholesterol. The recent cloning of the NPC1 and NPC2/HEJ genes, which are causative in NP-C disease, established the molecular basis for NP-C, but the functions of the NPC proteins have yet to be determined. The specific aims of this proposal will test the feasibility of using S. cerevisiae as a model system to study NPC1 function. The specific aims are: 1) to test the hypothesis that the S. cerevisiae homolog of NPC 1, NCR 1, is required for retrograde transport from the vacuole; and 2) to determine whether S. cerevisiae can be used as a model system to assess the functional consequences of patient mutations in the NPC1 gene. We will utilize fluorescently labeled lipids to test whether yeast cells lacking the NCR1 protein are defective in retrograde transport from the vacuole. To examine the functional consequences of patient mutations in NPC1, we will take advantage of a growth phenotype we have identified in yeast that lack a functional NCR1/NPC1 protein to assay for functional complementation. The health relatedness of this project is the establishment of a basis and possible future diagnostic tool for Niemann Pick disease type C.

Website: http://commons.cit.nih.gov/crisp3/CRISP.Generate_Ticket

- **Project Title: Biological Function of the Niemann Pick C Protein**

    Principal Investigator & Institution: Liscum, Laura; Professor; Physiology; Tufts University Boston 136 Harrison Ave Boston, Ma 02111

    Timing: Fiscal Year 2000; Project Start 1-MAY-1995; Project End 0-APR-2004

    Summary: Niemann-Pick type C (NPC) is an autosomal recessive lysosomal storage disease that causes progressive neurological degeneration in young children. Cultured NPC cells express defective transport of lipoprotein-derived cholesterol, resulting in lysosomal accumulation of cholesterol and aberrant regulation of cellular cholesterol homeostasis. The NPC1 gene was recently cloned. It encodes a 1245 aa membrane protein, with sequence homology to two proteins involved in cholesterol homeostasis. What is the biological function of NPC1? Our hypothesis is that NPC1 governs the targeting of cholesterol-carrying vesicles derived from lysosomes. We will test this hypothesis using wild-type and cholesterol transport defective Chinese hamster ovary cells. Specific im 1: To investigate the role of NPC1 in each cholesterol transport pathway. NPC1 will be expressed under the control of a regulated promoter; kinetics of cholesterol transport will be measured. Specific Aim 2: To determine if cellular cholesterol levels regulate NPC1. Transcriptional, translational and post- translational control of NPC1 expression by cellular cholesterol levels will be investigated. Specific Aim 3: To determine if the ced-1 gene is NPC1. Specific Aim 4: To analyze the intracellular location of NPC1. NPC1 distribution will be analyzed by density gradients and immunofluorescence microscopy. Specific Aim 5: To investigate the membrane orientation of NPC1. The domain organization of NPC1 will become important for structure/function analysis as disease-causing mutations are mapped. Knowledge of the biological function of NPC1 is critical for guiding the investigation into possible therapies for afflicted children. It also has relevance to the control of whole body cholesterol levels as well will gain information on the control of cholesterol availability for reverse cholesterol transport and bile acid metabolism.

    Website: http://commons.cit.nih.gov/crisp3/CRISP.Generate_Ticket

- **Project Title: Caveolar Function in Niemann-Pick Disease Type C**

    Principal Investigator & Institution: Heidenreich, Randall A.; Pediatrics; University of Arizona Tucson, Az 85721

Timing: Fiscal Year 2000; Project Start 5-MAR-1999; Project End 9-FEB-2004

Summary: Plasma membrane caveolae are specialized domains that have a central role in modulating intracellular cholesterol homeostasis. Alterations in the expression of caveolin-1, a cholesterol-binding proteins of caveolae, and accumulation of unesterified cholesterol within a caveolin-1 containing subcellular compartment, has been shown to occur within tissues and/or cultured cells derived from mice and humans with Niemann Pick type C (NPC). Our preliminary studies indicate that the NPC gene product (NPC1) is found in the detergent insoluble cellular fraction the same cellular fraction enriched in caveolae, implicating a direct relationship between NPC1 and caveolar function. Based on these observations, we believe that NPC is a unique and important model in which to define further the relationship between caveolae and intracellular cholesterol trafficking. The goals of this research project are to: 1) Determine if NPC1 is localized to caveolae. 2) Determine if cholesterol is enriched within caveolae isolated from NPC fibroblasts. 3) Determine the contribution of LDL-derived cholesterol and endogenously synthesized cholesterol to caveolae in NPC. 4) Determine if cholesterol efflux from caveolae from LDL-derived cholesterol and endogenously synthesized cholesterol to HDL is disrupted in NPC. 5) Determine the effects of disrupting caveolin-1 expression in heterozygous NPC cells on the trafficking of LDL-derived cholesterol and endogenously synthesized cholesterol to caveolae. These experiments will directly address the role of caveolae in cholesterol homeostasis as well as define the intracellular trafficking pathways utilized to regulate the removal of excess cholesterol mediated by HDL, an important process responsible for the preventing of atherosclerosis.

Website: http://commons.cit.nih.gov/crisp3/CRISP.Generate_Ticket

- **Project Title: Cellular Cholesterol Movement and Homeostatsis**

    Principal Investigator & Institution: Lange, Yvonne; Professor; Rush-Presbyterian-St Lukes Medical Ctr 1653 W Congress Pkwy Chicago, Il 60612

    Timing: Fiscal Year 2000; Project Start 1-JUN-1981; Project End 1-MAR-2003

    Summary: (Adapted from applicant's abstract): Cell cholesterol is of universal concern because of the enormous burden on health imposed by atherosclerotic cardiovascular disease. We now propose to continue our study o cellular cholesterol homeostasis. The hypothesis that the pool of cholesterol in the plasma membrane regulates its own abundance by signaling the endoplasmi reticulum (ER) through the regulated circulation of a stream of cholesterol will be tested. The set point of a putative cholesterol sensor in the plasma membrane will be characterized. The investigators will also test whether the cholesterol pool in the Golgi apparatus is regulated by the plasma membrane sensor; perhaps the Golgi serves as an intermediate in cholesterol transport. The flux of plasma membrane cholesterol through the lysosomes will be analyzed using cells from Niemann-Pick type C1 (NPC1) disease and cells treated with various amphiphiles which perturb cholesterol metabolism. The question of whether this movement represents specific transport or the flow of bulk plasma membrane bilayer will be addressed. The NPC1 gene product appears to be involved in cholesterol homeostasis. The investigators will analyze how its expression varies with cel cholesterol. Finally, the cell physiology of several sequenced mutants in NPC1 will be analyzed with respect to the gene defect to examine how NPC1 might function in cholesterol homeostasis.

Website: http://commons.cit.nih.gov/crisp3/CRISP.Generate_Ticket

- **Project Title: Experimental Pathology of Developing Nervous System**

  Principal Investigator & Institution: Suzuki, Kinuko L.; Professor of Pathology and Laboratory Me; Pathology and Lab Medicine; University of North Carolina Chapel Hill Box 2688, 910 Raleigh Rd Chapel Hill, Nc 27515

  Timing: Fiscal Year 2001; Project Start 1-MAY-1986; Project End 1-JUL-2005

  Summary: The ultimate goals of the investigations proposed in this application is to investigate the pathogenesis of the disease process and to explore therapeutic means of genetic neurodegenerative diseases, globoid cell leukodystrophy (GLD) and Niemann-Pick disease type C (NPC), using naturally occurring murine models, twitcher and NPC mice. GLD is a genetic demyelinating disease and formed myelin degenerates as result of apoptotic death of oligodendrocytes. NPC is a neurovisceral storage disease. Preliminary studies in our laboratory indicate apoptotic death of storage neurons and abnormal myelination suggesting problems in oligodendrocytes and/or oligodendrocyte progenitor cells. Chemokines/cytokines generated by cells within the CNS apparently play significant role(s) in pathogenesis of both diseases. In the murine model of GLD, twitcher mouse, massive infiltration of hematogenous lineage cells into the CNS is noted as a natural disease process. These cellular infiltrations appear to be regulated by pro-inflammatory cytokines and their inhibitors. In Aim 1, the mechanism of these cellular infiltration, role(s) of these hematogenous cells in the pathological process are investigated and also possible use of these cells as a vehicle to carry therapeutic gene in to the CNS will be explored. In Aim 2, oligodendrocyte progenitor cells will be investigated in twitcher CNS during demyelination as a natural disease process and during remyelination following bone marrow transplantation. The basic genetic defect of NPC is a defective intracellular transport of cholesterol. Cholesterol is an important lipid in normal neuronal maturation and myelination. Thus, in Aim 3, the underlying mechanism(s) of abnormal myelination and developmental pathological process will be investigated in NPC mouse. In NPC in humans as well as in mouse, neuronal storage is a very conspicuous pathology. Neuronal storage materials are thought to be largely glycolipid, ganglioside GM2. In the preliminary study, cholesterol accumulation has been demonstrated in neurons. So far defective transport of exogenous cholesterol has been demonstrated only in cultured NPC fibroblasts. We hypothesize that similar defect can be detected in neurons and in Aim 4, the hypothesis will be tested using cerebellar and/or hippocampal slice culture. Neurons in NPC die of apoptosis. Our preliminary studies have shown increasing expression of TNF-alphamRNA and intracellular proteins associated with death domain were upregulated, suggesting significant role of TNF-alpha in apoptotic neurodegeneration. Recent studies indicate that TNF-alpha promotes neurodegeneration through inhibition of survival signals activated by insulin-like growth factor receptor. Therefore, in Aim 5 possible protective role of insulin-like growth factor for neuronal degeneration will be tested by interbreeding NPC mouse with IGF-I transgenic mouse.

Website: http://commons.cit.nih.gov/crisp3/CRISP.Generate_Ticket

- **Project Title: Fluorescence-Based Studies of Sphingomyelin and Ceramide**

Principal Investigator & Institution: Schuchman, Edward H.; Professor; Human Genetics; Mount Sinai School of Medicine of Nyu of New York University New York, Ny 10029

Timing: Fiscal Year 2000; Project Start 1-SEP-2000; Project End 1-JUL-2003

Summary: This proposal seeks to extend research collaborations between the laboratories of Dr. Edward H. Schuchman in the Department of Human Genetics, Mount Sinai School of Medicine in NY, and Dr. Shimon Gatt, in the Department of Biochemistry, Hebrew University-Hadassah School of Medicine in Israel. The main aim is the development of novel approaches for studying the metabolism of two sphingolipids, sphingomyelin and ceramide, in normal cells and cells from patients with two genetic diseases, Niemann-Pick disease (due to acid sphingomyelinase [ASM] deficiency) and Farber disease (due to acid ceramidase [AC] deficiency), as well as the development of novel approaches for the treatment of these disorders. Fluorescence-based methods will be developed to determine whether pre-implantation stage embryos are affected with these diseases and/or to select normal sperm or eggs from carrier individuals for subsequent in vitro fertilization and prevention of the birth of affected children. This research relates to two funded NIH grants awarded to Dr. Schuchman, R01HD 28607, entitled "Acid Sphingomyelinase and Niemann-Pick Disease," and R01 DK 54830, entitled "Ceramidases, Ceramide, and Farber Disease" (estimated start date 12/1/99). R01 HD 28607 will serve as the parent grant for this research. Several approaches for the treatment of Niemann-Pick disease (NPD) will be developed. Aiming towards enzyme replacement therapy for NPD, ASM will be labeled with fluorescent probes and the trafficking (e.g., uptake, tissue distribution, etc) of the fluorescent enzyme will be monitored in cells and animals. Fluorescent ASM has already been prepared for these studies and shown to retain its catalytic activity using in vitro enzyme assay systems. Several novel approaches for treatment of NPD also will be studied: 1) inhibitors of sphingomyelin; 2) competitive of ASM will , aiming at protecting misfolded, mutant ASM from proteolysis; and 3) for improving enzyme replacement therapy for NPD, ASM will be modified in two ways: a) mannose will be linked to ASM, aiming at its increased uptake by the mannose receptor on microphages and Kupffer cells; and b) positively-charged (cationic) groups will be linked to ASM, aiming at its improved location within the lysosomes. Concordant with our efforts to develop therapy for NPD, studies will also be carried out to develop fluorescence-based methods to identify and select normal sperm or eggs from used for in vitro fertilization, preventing or remarkably diminishing the possibility of such barrier individuals having an affected child. For AC, reliable, fluorescence-based assays will continue to be developed, both for in vitro (i.e., using pure enzyme or extracts of cells and tissues), and in situ (i.e., in intact cells) analysis. Fluorescent procedures also will be used for selecting gene-modified cells which over-express AC, aiming at its purification, and inhibitors of AC and ceramide synthetase will be synthesized for evaluating the effects of increasing, or conversely, decreasing levels of cellular ceramide on the metabolism of sphingomyelin and glycolipids, as well as on cell viability.

Website: http://commons.cit.nih.gov/crisp3/CRISP.Generate_Ticket

- **Project Title: Hearing and Balance in Lysosomal Storage Diseases**

  Principal Investigator & Institution: Hennig, Anne K.; Medicine; Washington University Lindell and Skinker Blvd St. Louis, Mo 63130

Timing: Fiscal Year 2001; Project Start 1-MAY-2001; Project End 0-APR-2004

Summary: (provided by applicant): Progressive hearing loss is a common feature of many lysosomal storage diseases (LSDs). These diseases are usually caused by an inherited deficiency in the activity of one of the hydrolases that function within the lysosomes. As a result, partially degraded substrate accumulates within lysosomes, causing a progressive impairment of cellular and organ function. The hearing loss is usually mixed; the conductive component can be accounted for by ossicle malformation, incomplete pneumatization and chronic otitis media, but the mechanisms underlying the sensorineural component are unknown. Furthermore, vestibular function has been examined only in patients with Fabry disease. Since effective therapies are now being developed for many of the LSDs, it is crucial to understand the otological manifestations of this group of diseases and the impact of these therapies on the underlying middle and inner ear defects. I propose to determine the extent and immediate cause(s) of hearing and vestibular dysfunction in six mouse models of different LSDs: MPS I/Hurler, MPS II/Hunter, MPS IIIB/Sanfilippo B, MPS VII/Sly, Fabry, and Niemann- Pick A/B. All of the human counterparts have associated hearing loss except Niemann-Pick A/B. Since these diseases all share impaired degradation of the carbohydrate component of cell-surface and extracellular macromolecules, the findings of this study will provide insights to potentially common mechanisms underlying the hearing and vestibular dysfunction in LSDs. In addition, virus- mediated gene transfer studies already in progress in MPS VII mice will be extended to examine the effects of therapy on the middle and inner ear. These studies will lay the groundwork for designing rational treatment therapies that will preserve or improve hearing and vestibular function. The specific aims of this application are: (1) to determine the extent and progression of hearing deficits in six mouse models of lysosomal storage diseases; (2) to determine the extent and progression of balance deficits in these mouse models; and (3) to determine the efficacy of gene therapy in correcting structural and functional deficits contributing to hearing and balance disturbances in MPS VII mice, a prototype LSD model.

Website: http://commons.cit.nih.gov/crisp3/CRISP.Generate_Ticket

- **Project Title: Mechanisms of Tau-Based Neurodegeneration**

Principal Investigator & Institution: Forman, Mark S.; Pathology and Lab Medicine; University of Pennsylvania 3451 Walnut Philadelphia, Pa 19104

Timing: Fiscal Year 2001; Project Start 0-SEP-2001; Project End 1-AUG-2006

Summary: Filamentous tau inclusions in neurons, astrocytes and oligodendrocytes are the neuropathological hallmark of both sporadic and familial tauopathies. Alzheimer's disease (AD), the most common tauopathy, is characterized by the deposition of numerous Ap-rich senile plaques as well as neurofibrillary tangles composed of hyperphosphorylated tau in the brains of affected individuals. Compelling evidence in support of the hypothesis for a causative role of tau in neurodegeneration is provided by the studies of tauopathies other than AD, which demonstrate abundant filamentous pathology in the absence of extracellular amyloid deposition. Furthermore, the identification of pathogenic tau gene mutations in familial tauopathies, termed frontotemporal dementia with parkinsonism linked to chromosome 17, provided unequivocal support for the hypothesis that defects in the tau gene alone are sufficient to cause neurodegeneration. These tau gene mutations are pathogenic because they perturb alternative splicing, alter the biophysical properties and/or affect the microtubule binding function of tau. However, it remains unclear why in both sporadic and familial tauopathies there is selective degeneration of specific subsets of neurons and glia. To test the hypothesis that additional genetic or epigenetic perturbations that alter the expression, function or biochemical properties of the tau protein lead to distinct topographic and cell-type specific neurodegeneration, the following specific aims are proposed: 1) An analysis of cell-type specific differences in the expression and biochemical properties of tau in brain tissue form both sporadic and familial tauopathies. 2) Development of transgenic mice that overexpress human wild type or mutant tau utilizing promoters that drive expression in specific cell lineages. The development of tau pathology in the specific cell types will be assessed morphologically and biochemically. 3) Determine mechanisms of tau-mediated neurodegeneration in primary cultures of neurons, astrocytes and oligodendrocytes derived from the brains of the transgenic animals developed in Aim 2. These studies will provide invaluable information on the pathogenesis of filamentous tau inclusions in the specific cell lineages within the brain, thus providing insight into the phenotypic expression of tauopathies. The successful generation of animal models will accelerate future research to discover new techniques for the diagnosis and treatment of tauopathies, including AD, the most dementing illness characterized by prominent tau pathology. This proposal will also facilitate my transition from a trainee to a fully independent experimental neuropathologist.

Website: http://commons.cit.nih.gov/crisp3/CRISP.Generate_Ticket

- **Project Title: Neurosteroidogenesis in Niemann-Pick Type C Disease**

    Principal Investigator & Institution: Griffin, Lisa D.; Neurology; University of California San Francisco 500 Parnassus Ave San Francisco, Ca 94122

    Timing: Fiscal Year 2000; Project Start 3-JUL-1997; Project End 0-JUN-2002

    Summary: The proposed development award focuses on the role of neurosteriods in Niemann-Pick type C disease as well as the developing rodent nervous system. The candidate's research background is in biochemical genetics and molecular biology with long term interest in molecular developmental neurobiology. Immediate goals during the period of this research award include the accumulation of experience in basic neurobiological research techniques as well as a greater understanding of neural systems and steroid biology as a whole, serving as an outstanding complement for the candidate's previous research training in molecular genetics. Long term goals are to apply both of these areas of experience to a research and clinical career in molecular and developmental neurobiology. It has recently been shown that specific types of steroid hormones, called neurosteroids, are synthesized de novo in the brain using the same steroid synthesizing enzymes found in the adrenal and gonads. These neurosteroids, have profound effects on the modulation of ion influx through the GABAA and NMDA receptors and have been also shown to affect embryonal neuronal and glial survival and differentiation in culture. The role of these neurosteriods in the development of the normal nervous system are unknown. This proposal seeks to investigate the alterations in neurosteriods in the nervous system of the murine model of Niemann Pick type C (NP- C) through analysis of endogenous neurosteroids in neural cell culture and in the developing rodent. The role of neurosteroids in neuronal demise will be examined through analysis of dendritic growth and regression. The factors that influence expression of the steroidogenic enzymes and the effects of neurosteriods on cortical growth and differentiation will be determined. This information will be used to create mouse models with abnormal neurosteriod synthesis to determine specific effects on behavior, neuronal excitation, and neuronal network formation. These experiments will provide vital information about the role of neurosteriods in the generation of the NP-C phenotype.

    Website: http://commons.cit.nih.gov/crisp3/CRISP.Generate_Ticket

- **Project Title: Niemann-Pick C and Intracellular Cholesterol Transport**

    Principal Investigator & Institution: Ioannou, Yiannis A.; Associate Professor of Human Molecular m; Human Genetics; Mount Sinai School of Medicine of Nyu of New York University New York, Ny 10029

    Timing: Fiscal Year 2000; Project Start 1-JUN-2000; Project End 0-APR-2005

    Summary: The overall objective of the proposed research is to investigate the mechanisms of intracellular cholesterol transport, especially cholesterol egress from the endosome/lysosome. These studies will exploit the experiment of nature, NPC disease, in which at least two different defective genes impair cholesterol egress and result in endosomal/lysosomal cholesterol accumulation and a neurodegenerative phenotype. Recently, the NPC1 gene on chromosome 18 was isolated by positional cloning. The 4.5 kb cDNA encodes a novel 1278 residue polypeptide with several putative membrane spanning regions, which presumably is involved in cholesterol transport (e.g. transporter, pump, docking protein, etc.). Initial studies will determine the subcellular location and topology o the wild-type NPC1 protein. Immunohistochemistry and immunoelectron microscopy using monoclonal and polyclonal antibodies will be used to define the subcellular location of NPC1. The cytosolic or lumenal topology of the five NPC1-predicted hydrophilic loops will be assessed by expression and analysis of a series of NPC1 cDNAs with flag-tags in each of the loops. Our results indicate that the sterol- sensing domain (SSD) of NPC1 is in the same orientation as in HMG-CoA reductase and SCAP, whose topologies are known. The significance of the NPC1 SSD will be further evaluated. In addition, our studies indicate that loop "c" is functionally significant, as constructs containing a FLAG sequence in this loop fail to complement NPC fibroblasts. To identify structure/function relationships, putative functional domains will be expressed and their potential inhibitory effects on the endogenous protein will be assessed. These studies should enhance our understanding of subcellular cholesterol transport and metabolism and provide insights into the pathogenesis of NPC disease. We should emphasize that we have already made significant contributions in the subcellular location (defined the location of NPC1 as the late endosome and not lysosomes) and topology determination of NPC1 (solved the complete topology of this polytopic glycoprotein) and have identified a novel protein targeting motif, a functional domain of NPC1 and a potential 85 kDa protein that associates with NPC1.

    Website: http://commons.cit.nih.gov/crisp3/CRISP.Generate_Ticket

- **Project Title: Niemann-Pick Disease**

  Principal Investigator & Institution: Wasserstein, Melissa P.; General Clinical Research Ctr; Mount Sinai School of Medicine of Nyu of New York University New York, Ny 10029

  Timing: Fiscal Year 2001; Project Start 1-MAY-2001; Project End 0-APR-2006

  Summary: Types A and B Niemann-Pick disease (NPD) are lysosomal storage disorders caused by deficient acid sphingomyelinase (ASM). Type A NPD is a severe neurodegenerative disease of infancy that typically causes death by three years of age. Type B NPD is characterized by the lack of neurological involvement and a phenotypic spectrum ranging from severe multisystem disease and early demise, to a milder condition of adulthood. The principal manifestations of Type B NPD include infiltrative pulmonary disease, hepatosplenomegaly, hyperlipidemia, and growth retardation and delayed puberty in children. The difficulty in differentiating between Types A and B NPD early in the disease course limits prognostic information, complicates family planning, and interferes with the selection of candidates for early therapeutic endeavors. Therefore, the ability to predict disease severity using information derived from empiric correlations between genotype and phenotype would be of significant value. Treatment for Types A and B NPD is primarily supportive, although bone marrow transplantation has been attempted with very limited success in Type B NPD patients. The therapeutic success of enzyme replacement therapy (ERT) in a related lysosomal storage disorder, Type I Gaucher disease, coupled with the demonstrated effectiveness of ERT in the Niemann-Pick mouse, provide the rationale for a clinical trial using recombinant ASM in patients with non-neuronopathic Type B NPD. The proposed studies will therefore focus on determining correlations between the clinical, radiographic and biochemical manifestations of Types A and B NPD and specific ASM mutations. In addition, the safety and effectiveness of ERT for Type B NPD will be evaluated. Thus the specific aims of the proposed research are: 1) to determine the natural history of Types A and B NPD and identify causative ASM mutations for genotype/phenotype correlations and 2) to evaluate the role of ERT for Type B NPD. An FDA-approved phase I/II clinical trial will be performed in Type B NPD patients to determine the safety and effectiveness of varying doses of intravenously administered recombinant human ASM. A series of clinical, biochemical, and pharmacological studies will be performed in order to evaluate the therapeutic effectiveness as well as the pharmacokinetics of the drug. In sum, these studies should provide important diagnostic and therapeutic information to improve the outcome of patients diagnosed with NPD.

Website: http://commons.cit.nih.gov/crisp3/CRISP.Generate_Ticket

- **Project Title: Non Invasive Monitoring of NPC C Progression and Therapy**

  Principal Investigator & Institution: Gillies, Robert J.; Professor; Biochemistry; University of Arizona Tucson, Az 85721

  Timing: Fiscal Year 2001; Project Start 2-APR-2001; Project End 1-MAR-2002

  Summary: (Verbatim from Applicant's Abstract): The overall goal of this research is to develop a non-invasive and quantitative method to monitor progression of NP-C disease and its response to successful therapy. Niemann-Pick type C disease (NP-C) is an inheritable defect in intracellular cholesterol trafficking with a gene frequency of 1:200. Although it is rare, the defect is particularly devastating because most NP-C suffers present in early childhood with progressive ataxia, leading to death before puberty. The major gene responsible for NP-C was identified in 1997, and its structure lends some clues as to its cellular biochemical function. Investigating the molecular mechanisms underlying this disease is leading to development of rational therapies. Development of therapies is also being helped with a NP-C mouse model. A major problem is that current therapeutic endpoints are limited to qualitative measures of neurological response patterns or delayed onset of death. These endpoints are far from ideal since they are neither sensitive nor quantitative. A sensitive, reliable and quantitative method to monitor progression of NP-C and regression in response to successful therapy is needed. Magnetic Resonance Imaging (MRI) has great potential to provide such a method because it is non-invasive, it is equally applicable to animal models and to human patients, and it can generate data which are quantifiably sensitive to changes in NP-C. Since MRI analyses are non-invasive, therapeutic responses can be benchmarked against the subjects' own background, and this increases the sensitivity of measurement several fold. Because MRI methods are applicable to animal models and human patients, methods developed for monitoring NP-C in mice can be translated rapidly to the human patient population. The goal of this research is to develop MRI methods to monitor NP-C that are sensitive, reliable and quantitative. Such methods will hasten the development and application of rational therapies and improve treatment of human patients. The approach to this goal will involve quantitatively relating the MR-visible parameters to the progression of the disease, defined using neurological, biochemical and histological markers. MR techniques to be investigated are magnetization transfer contrast (MTC) imaging and diffusion imaging (DI). Preliminary data indicate that these modalities can successfully discriminate NP-C mice from normal littermates. The two major organ systems to be investigated are the brain and liver, since these are greatly affected in clinical disease. These methods will then be used to monitor the progression of NP-C disease in individual homozygous NP-C mice and those undergoing experimental therapies. A direct outcome of this project will be the development of quantitative and reliable methods, which can be exported to other labs for animal work, or to clinical centers for analyses of human patients. We will continue to work with other NP-C researchers to either analyze their animals undergoing therapy or to help them apply these methods at their institutions.

Website: http://commons.cit.nih.gov/crisp3/CRISP.Generate_Ticket

- **Project Title: Novel Approaches to Niemann-Pick Type C Disease**

    Principal Investigator & Institution: Maue, Robert A.; Physiology; Dartmouth College Hanover, Nh 03755

    Timing: Fiscal Year 2002; Project Start 5-DEC-2001; Project End 0-NOV-2004

    Summary: (Provided By Applicant): Despite recent identification of a gene (npc1) that is mutated in Niemann- Pick Type C (NPC) disease, little is known about the mechanism(s) by which this error leads to the devastating, neurodegenerative changes and childhood neuropathology characteristic of this disorder. We recently provided new insight into the functional implications of this mutation by showing that neurons from the brain of embryonic mice, with NPC disease (npc/nih mice), exhibit not only abnormal cholesterol metabolism, but also deficient morphological and biochemical responses to the neurotrophin, BDNF. In additional experiments, we found that the insensitivity to BDNF stems from a lack of TrkB activation, despite expression of these receptors on the cell surface. Guided by these results, we propose to extend and expand our analysis of this disorder. First, we will define further the nature and extent of the defects in neuronal membrane signaling in NPC disease. We will evaluate the morphological responses to other growth factors, and use cell fractionation and gradient centrifugation to determine if the localization of TrkB and other growth factor receptors to low density, cholesterol-enriched microdomains ("lipid rafts") in the plasma membrane is disrupted in neurons from npc/nih mice. Western blot analysis will also be used to assay the distribution of signaling intermediates often found in lipid rafts, such as Ras and Src, as well as the distribution of the GM1, GM2, and GM3 gangliosides which, in some cases, exhibit altered expression in NPC disease, and in other studies have been shown to be localized to lipid rafts and influence growth factor receptor function. The influence of NPC disease on membrane signaling, through ion channels and synaptic connections, will also be assessed using patch clamp measures of spontaneous activity, evoked activity, and synaptic currents in Purkinje cells in slices of the cerebellum, a region our in situ hybridization studies indicate express high-levels of the npc1 gene. Second, we will test the potential of adenoviral-mediated approaches to retard, halt, or even reverse the neurological deficits observed in NPC disease. To begin, we will determine if viral-mediated expression of an Npc1/GFP fusion protein can restore cholesterol metabolism and BDNF responsiveness to cultured striatal neurons from npc/nih mice. Furthermore, using different modes of infection, including intravenous administration and direct injection into the brain of npc/nih mice, we will assess the extent and duration of Npc1/GFP expression in vivo using confocal microscopic analysis of brain sections, and determine if viral-mediated expression influences aspects of physiology and behavior compromised in NPC disease, including weight, life-span, reproductive capacity, and motor performance. The proposed studies represent novel ideas and approaches with regard to NPC disease, and will both increase our understanding of the neurological deficits that occur and explore a potential therapeutic strategy for what is, at present, an incurable disorder.

Website: http://commons.cit.nih.gov/crisp3/CRISP.Generate_Ticket

- **Project Title: Synaptic Mechnisms in Drosophila Neurodegeneration Model**

  Principal Investigator & Institution: Broadie, Kendal S.; Biology; University of Utah 200 S University St Salt Lake City, Ut 84112

  Timing: Fiscal Year 2001; Project Start 1-MAY-2001; Project End 0-APR-2005

  Summary: Description (Provided by applicant): The hypothesis driving this proposal is that presynaptic dysfunction is a common causative factor leading to cell death in multiple inherited neurodegenerative diseases. This hypothesis is based on the observations that 1) synaptic function mediates neuronal survival during development, 2) mutations which strongly impair presynaptic function result in massive, progressive neuronal degeneration, 3) a number of presynaptic proteins have been directly implicated in neurodegenerative diseases and 4) neuronal dysfunction/synapse loss is known to precede by a substantial period the manifestation of cell death in these diseases. To date, however, there is no established direct evidence of synaptic dysfunction mediating neuronal death during neurodegenerative disease states. The goal of this proposal is to assay synaptic maintenance in two genetic models of neurodegenerative diseases: Drosophila models of Parkinson's Disease (PD), a classic "protein storage" disease, and Niemann-Pick Type C (NP-C), a classic "lipid storage" disease. Drosophila was selected for its attractive properties as a new molecular genetic model of neurodegeneration, and its long history as the foremost genetic model for synaptic studies. PD and NP-C were selected as representative of a large number of related neurodegenerative disorders. The Drosophila PD model has been recently established through transgenic over-expression of human alpha-synuclein (a presynaptic protein) and shown to accurately recapitulate the diagnostic features of human PD. A Drosophila model of NP-C is being established through mutation (loss-of-function) of the endogenous NPC I gene, the known cause of human NP-C disease. Specifically, this proposal is to conduct age-progressive studies of synaptic mechanisms in Drosophila PD and NP-C models to correlate synaptic maintenance with the onset, progression and prevalence of neurodegeneration. The first aim is to improve Drosophila models by generating fluorescently tagged alpha-synuclein and NPCI proteins whose levels can be reversibly regulated through a temperature-dependent ubiquination strategy. Secondly, to confirm gross features of neurodegeneration in these models with behavioral assays and examination of nervous system/neuronal architecture. Third, and most importantly, to assay synaptic development, function and maintenance in these models. Assays will include electrophysiological measurements of neurotransmission, quantitative fluorescent optical imaging of protein and lipid dynamics in the presynaptic terminal and ultrastructural studies of presynaptic architecture. Together, these studies will allow a conclusive determination of whether synaptic maintenance is compromised in PD and NP-C, and is the causative factor that leads to neuronal cell death and neurodegeneration in these disease states.

Website: http://commons.cit.nih.gov/crisp3/CRISP.Generate_Ticket

E-Journals: PubMed Central[19]

PubMed Central (PMC) is a digital archive of life sciences journal literature developed and managed by the National Center for Biotechnology

---

[19] Adapted from the National Library of Medicine: http://www.pubmedcentral.nih.gov/about/intro.html.

Information (NCBI) at the U.S. National Library of Medicine (NLM).[20] Access to this growing archive of e-journals is free and unrestricted.[21] To search, go to **http://www.pubmedcentral.nih.gov/index.html#search**, and type "Niemann-Pick disease" (or synonyms) into the search box. This search gives you access to full-text articles. The following is a sample of items found for Niemann-Pick disease in the PubMed Central database:

- **Accumulation of cholera toxin and GM1 ganglioside in the early endosome of Niemann--Pick C1-deficient cells** by Yuko Sugimoto, Haruaki Ninomiya, Yuki Ohsaki, Katsumi Higaki, Joanna P. Davies, Yiannis A. Ioannou, and Kousaku Ohno; 2001 October 23
  http://www.pubmedcentral.nih.gov/articlerender.fcgi?artid=60064

- **Cessation of rapid late endosomal tubulovesicular trafficking in Niemann--Pick type C1 disease** by Mei Zhang, Nancy K. Dwyer, Dona C. Love, Adele Cooney, Marcy Comly, Edward Neufeld, Peter G. Pentchev, E. Joan Blanchette-Mackie, and John A. Hanover; 2001 April 10
  http://www.pubmedcentral.nih.gov/articlerender.fcgi?artid=31858

- **Cholesterol accumulation in tissues of the Niemann-Pick type C mouse is determined by the rate of lipoprotein-cholesterol uptake through the coated-pit pathway in each organ** by Chonglun Xie, Stephen D. Turley, and John M. Dietschy; 1999 October 12
  http://www.pubmedcentral.nih.gov/articlerender.fcgi?artid=18400

- **Dynamic Movements of Organelles Containing Niemann-Pick C1 Protein: NPC1 Involvement in Late Endocytic Events** by Dennis C. Ko, Michael D. Gordon, Janet Y. Jin, and Matthew P. Scott; 2001 March
  http://www.pubmedcentral.nih.gov/articlerender.fcgi?artid=30967

- **Linkage of Niemann-Pick Disease Type C to Human Chromosome 18** by ED Carstea, MH Polymeropoulos, CC Parker, SD Detera-Wadleigh, RR O'Neill, MC Paterson, E Goldin, H Xiao, RE Straub, MT Vanier, RO Brady, and PG Pentchev; 1993 March 1
  http://www.pubmedcentral.nih.gov/articlerender.fcgi?rendertype=abstract&artid=46008

- **Localization of Niemann--Pick C1 protein in astrocytes: Implications for neuronal degeneration in Niemann -- Pick type C disease** by Shutish C. Patel, Sundar Suresh, Ujendra Kumar, C. Y. Hu, Adele Cooney, E. Joan

---

[20] With PubMed Central, NCBI is taking the lead in preservation and maintenance of open access to electronic literature, just as NLM has done for decades with printed biomedical literature. PubMed Central aims to become a world-class library of the digital age.

[21] The value of PubMed Central, in addition to its role as an archive, lies the availability of data from diverse sources stored in a common format in a single repository. Many journals already have online publishing operations, and there is a growing tendency to publish material online only, to the exclusion of print.

Blanchette-Mackie, Edward B. Neufeld, Ramesh C. Patel, Roscoe O. Brady, Yogesh C. Patel, Peter G. Pentchev, and Wei-Yi Ong; 1999 February 16
http://www.pubmedcentral.nih.gov/articlerender.fcgi?artid=15549

- **Niemann-Pick C1 protein: Obligatory roles for N-terminal domains and lysosomal targeting in cholesterol mobilization** by Hidemichi Watari, E. Joan Blanchette-Mackie, Nancy K. Dwyer, Jane M. Glick, Shutish Patel, Edward B. Neufeld, Roscoe O. Brady, Peter G. Pentchev, and Jerome F. Strauss, III; 1999 February 2
http://www.pubmedcentral.nih.gov/articlerender.fcgi?artid=15306

The National Library of Medicine: PubMed

One of the quickest and most comprehensive ways to find academic studies in both English and other languages is to use PubMed, maintained by the National Library of Medicine. The advantage of PubMed over previously mentioned sources is that it covers a greater number of domestic and foreign references. It is also free to the public.[22] If the publisher has a Web site that offers full text of its journals, PubMed will provide links to that site, as well as to sites offering other related data. User registration, a subscription fee, or some other type of fee may be required to access the full text of articles in some journals.

To generate your own bibliography of studies dealing with Niemann-Pick disease, simply go to the PubMed Web site at **www.ncbi.nlm.nih.gov/pubmed**. Type "Niemann-Pick disease" (or synonyms) into the search box, and click "Go."

Vocabulary Builder

Aberrant: Wandering or deviating from the usual or normal course. [EU]

Assay: Determination of the amount of a particular constituent of a mixture, or of the biological or pharmacological potency of a drug. [EU]

Bile: An emulsifying agent produced in the liver and secreted into the

---

[22] PubMed was developed by the National Center for Biotechnology Information (NCBI) at the National Library of Medicine (NLM) at the National Institutes of Health (NIH). The PubMed database was developed in conjunction with publishers of biomedical literature as a search tool for accessing literature citations and linking to full-text journal articles at Web sites of participating publishers. Publishers that participate in PubMed supply NLM with their citations electronically prior to or at the time of publication.

duodenum. Its composition includes bile acids and salts, cholesterol, and electrolytes. It aids digestion of fats in the duodenum. [NIH]

Biosynthesis: The building up of a chemical compound in the physiologic processes of a living organism. [EU]

Carbohydrate: An aldehyde or ketone derivative of a polyhydric alcohol, particularly of the pentahydric and hexahydric alcohols. They are so named because the hydrogen and oxygen are usually in the proportion to form water, (CH2O)n. The most important carbohydrates are the starches, sugars, celluloses, and gums. They are classified into mono-, di-, tri-, poly- and heterosaccharides. [EU]

Cardiovascular: Pertaining to the heart and blood vessels. [EU]

Cerebellar: Pertaining to the cerebellum. [EU]

Cerebellum: Part of the metencephalon that lies in the posterior cranial fossa behind the brain stem. It is concerned with the coordination of movement. [NIH]

Cholera: An acute diarrheal disease endemic in India and Southeast Asia whose causative agent is vibrio cholerae. This condition can lead to severe dehydration in a matter of hours unless quickly treated. [NIH]

Chronic: Persisting over a long period of time. [EU]

Cortical: Pertaining to or of the nature of a cortex or bark. [EU]

Cytokines: Non-antibody proteins secreted by inflammatory leukocytes and some non-leukocytic cells, that act as intercellular mediators. They differ from classical hormones in that they are produced by a number of tissue or cell types rather than by specialized glands. They generally act locally in a paracrine or autocrine rather than endocrine manner. [NIH]

Dementia: An acquired organic mental disorder with loss of intellectual abilities of sufficient severity to interfere with social or occupational functioning. The dysfunction is multifaceted and involves memory, behavior, personality, judgment, attention, spatial relations, language, abstract thought, and other executive functions. The intellectual decline is usually progressive, and initially spares the level of consciousness. [NIH]

Dendritic: 1. branched like a tree. 2. pertaining to or possessing dendrites. [EU]

Diffusion: The process of becoming diffused, or widely spread; the spontaneous movement of molecules or other particles in solution, owing to their random thermal motion, to reach a uniform concentration throughout the solvent, a process requiring no addition of energy to the system. [EU]

Drosophila: A genus of small, two-winged flies containing approximately 900 described species. These organisms are the most extensively studied of all genera from the standpoint of genetics and cytology. [NIH]

Electrophysiological: Pertaining to electrophysiology, that is a branch of physiology that is concerned with the electric phenomena associated with living bodies and involved in their functional activity. [EU]

Embryo: In animals, those derivatives of the fertilized ovum that eventually become the offspring, during their period of most rapid development, i.e., after the long axis appears until all major structures are represented. In man, the developing organism is an embryo from about two weeks after fertilization to the end of seventh or eighth week. [EU]

Empiric: Empirical; depending upon experience or observation alone, without using scientific method or theory. [EU]

Excitation: An act of irritation or stimulation or of responding to a stimulus; the addition of energy, as the excitation of a molecule by absorption of photons. [EU]

Exogenous: Developed or originating outside the organism, as exogenous disease. [EU]

Fibroblasts: Connective tissue cells which secrete an extracellular matrix rich in collagen and other macromolecules. [NIH]

Genotype: The genetic constitution of the individual; the characterization of the genes. [NIH]

Gonads: The gamete-producing glands, ovary or testis. [NIH]

Homeostasis: A tendency to stability in the normal body states (internal environment) of the organism. It is achieved by a system of control mechanisms activated by negative feedback; e.g. a high level of carbon dioxide in extracellular fluid triggers increased pulmonary ventilation, which in turn causes a decrease in carbon dioxide concentration. [EU]

Hormones: Chemical substances having a specific regulatory effect on the activity of a certain organ or organs. The term was originally applied to substances secreted by various endocrine glands and transported in the bloodstream to the target organs. It is sometimes extended to include those substances that are not produced by the endocrine glands but that have similar effects. [NIH]

Hybridization: The genetic process of crossbreeding to produce a hybrid. Hybrid nucleic acids can be formed by nucleic acid hybridization of DNA and RNA molecules. Protein hybridization allows for hybrid proteins to be formed from polypeptide chains. [NIH]

Hydrophilic: Readily absorbing moisture; hygroscopic; having strongly polar groups that readily interact with water. [EU]

Hyperlipidemia: An excess of lipids in the blood. [NIH]

Immunohistochemistry: Histochemical localization of immunoreactive substances using labeled antibodies as reagents. [NIH]

Implantation: The insertion or grafting into the body of biological, living, inert, or radioactive material. [EU]

Infiltration: The diffusion or accumulation in a tissue or cells of substances not normal to it or in amounts of the normal. Also, the material so accumulated. [EU]

Insulin: A protein hormone secreted by beta cells of the pancreas. Insulin plays a major role in the regulation of glucose metabolism, generally promoting the cellular utilization of glucose. It is also an important regulator of protein and lipid metabolism. Insulin is used as a drug to control insulin-dependent diabetes mellitus. [NIH]

Invasive: 1. having the quality of invasiveness. 2. involving puncture or incision of the skin or insertion of an instrument or foreign material into the body; said of diagnostic techniques. [EU]

Kinetic: Pertaining to or producing motion. [EU]

Lipoprotein: Any of the lipid-protein complexes in which lipids are transported in the blood; lipoprotein particles consist of a spherical hydrophobic core of triglycerides or cholesterol esters surrounded by an amphipathic monolayer of phospholipids, cholesterol, and apolipoproteins; the four principal classes are high-density, low-density, and very-low-density lipoproteins and chylomicrons. [EU]

Localization: 1. the determination of the site or place of any process or lesion. 2. restriction to a circumscribed or limited area. 3. prelocalization. [EU]

Malformation: A morphologic defect resulting from an intrinsically abnormal developmental process. [EU]

Microscopy: The application of microscope magnification to the study of materials that cannot be properly seen by the unaided eye. [NIH]

Neuronal: Pertaining to a neuron or neurons (= conducting cells of the nervous system). [EU]

Neurons: The basic cellular units of nervous tissue. Each neuron consists of a body, an axon, and dendrites. Their purpose is to receive, conduct, and transmit impulses in the nervous system. [NIH]

Nickel: Nickel. A trace element with the atomic symbol Ni, atomic number 28, and atomic weight 58.69. It is a cofactor of the enzyme urease. [NIH]

Organelles: Specific particles of membrane-bound organized living substances present in eukaryotic cells, such as the mitochondria; the golgi apparatus; endoplasmic reticulum; lysomomes; plastids; and vacuoles. [NIH]

Ossicle: A small bone. [EU]

Otitis: Inflammation of the ear, which may be marked by pain, fever, abnormalities of hearing, hearing loss, tinnitus, and vertigo. [EU]

Ovary: Either of the paired glands in the female that produce the female germ cells and secrete some of the female sex hormones. [NIH]

Parkinsonism: A group of neurological disorders characterized by hypokinesia, tremor, and muscular rigidity. [EU]

Pediatrics: A medical specialty concerned with maintaining health and providing medical care to children from birth to adolescence. [NIH]

Pharmacokinetics: The action of drugs in the body over a period of time, including the processes of absorption, distribution, localization in tissues, biotransformation, and excretion. [EU]

Phenotype: The outward appearance of the individual. It is the product of interactions between genes and between the genotype and the environment. This includes the killer phenotype, characteristic of yeasts. [NIH]

Polypeptide: A peptide which on hydrolysis yields more than two amino acids; called tripeptides, tetrapeptides, etc. according to the number of amino acids contained. [EU]

Presynaptic: Situated proximal to a synapse, or occurring before the synapse is crossed. [EU]

Prevalence: The total number of cases of a given disease in a specified population at a designated time. It is differentiated from incidence, which refers to the number of new cases in the population at a given time. [NIH]

Proteins: Polymers of amino acids linked by peptide bonds. The specific sequence of amino acids determines the shape and function of the protein. [NIH]

Puberty: The period during which the secondary sex characteristics begin to develop and the capability of sexual reproduction is attained. [EU]

Receptor: 1. a molecular structure within a cell or on the surface characterized by (1) selective binding of a specific substance and (2) a specific physiologic effect that accompanies the binding, e.g., cell-surface receptors for peptide hormones, neurotransmitters, antigens, complement fragments, and immunoglobulins and cytoplasmic receptors for steroid hormones. 2. a sensory nerve terminal that responds to stimuli of various kinds. [EU]

Recombinant: 1. a cell or an individual with a new combination of genes not found together in either parent; usually applied to linked genes. [EU]

Retrograde: 1. moving backward or against the usual direction of flow. 2. degenerating, deteriorating, or catabolic. [EU]

Saccharomyces: A genus of ascomycetous fungi of the family Saccharomycetaceae, order saccharomycetales. [NIH]

Serum: The clear portion of any body fluid; the clear fluid moistening serous membranes. 2. blood serum; the clear liquid that separates from blood on clotting. 3. immune serum; blood serum from an immunized animal used for passive immunization; an antiserum; antitoxin, or antivenin. [EU]

Spectrum: A charted band of wavelengths of electromagnetic vibrations obtained by refraction and diffraction. By extension, a measurable range of activity, such as the range of bacteria affected by an antibiotic (antibacterial s.) or the complete range of manifestations of a disease. [EU]

Sporadic: Neither endemic nor epidemic; occurring occasionally in a random or isolated manner. [EU]

Substrate: A substance upon which an enzyme acts. [EU]

Synaptic: Pertaining to or affecting a synapse (= site of functional apposition between neurons, at which an impulse is transmitted from one neuron to another by electrical or chemical means); pertaining to synapsis (= pairing off in point-for-point association of homologous chromosomes from the male and female pronuclei during the early prophase of meiosis). [EU]

Toxin: A poison; frequently used to refer specifically to a protein produced by some higher plants, certain animals, and pathogenic bacteria, which is highly toxic for other living organisms. Such substances are differentiated from the simple chemical poisons and the vegetable alkaloids by their high molecular weight and antigenicity. [EU]

Vestibular: Pertaining to or toward a vestibule. In dental anatomy, used to refer to the tooth surface directed toward the vestibule of the mouth. [EU]

CHAPTER 5. BOOKS ON NIEMANN-PICK DISEASE

Overview

This chapter provides bibliographic book references relating to Niemann-Pick disease. You have many options to locate books on Niemann-Pick disease. The simplest method is to go to your local bookseller and inquire about titles that they have in stock or can special order for you. Some parents, however, prefer online sources (e.g. **www.amazon.com** and **www.bn.com**). In addition to online booksellers, excellent sources for book titles on Niemann-Pick disease include the Combined Health Information Database and the National Library of Medicine. Once you have found a title that interests you, visit your local public or medical library to see if it is available for loan.

Book Summaries: Online Booksellers

Commercial Internet-based booksellers, such as Amazon.com and Barnes & Noble.com, offer summaries which have been supplied by each title's publisher. Some summaries also include customer reviews. Your local bookseller may have access to in-house and commercial databases that index all published books (e.g. Books in Print®).

The National Library of Medicine Book Index

The National Library of Medicine at the National Institutes of Health has a massive database of books published on healthcare and biomedicine. Go to the following Internet site, **http://locatorplus.gov/**, and then select "Search LOCATORplus." Once you are in the search area, simply type "Niemann-

Pick disease" (or synonyms) into the search box, and select "books only." From there, results can be sorted by publication date, author, or relevance. The following was recently catalogued by the National Library of Medicine:[23]

- **Pick's disease and Pick complex.** Author: edited by Andrew Kertesz, David G. Munoz; Year: 1998; New York: Wiley-Liss Inc., c1998; ISBN: 047117792X (cloth: alk. paper)
  http://www.amazon.com/exec/obidos/ASIN/047117792X/icongroupinterna

Chapters on Niemann-Pick Disease

Frequently, Niemann-Pick disease will be discussed within a book, perhaps within a specific chapter. In order to find chapters that are specifically dealing with Niemann-Pick disease, an excellent source of abstracts is the Combined Health Information Database. You will need to limit your search to book chapters and Niemann-Pick disease using the "Detailed Search" option. Go to the following hyperlink: **http://chid.nih.gov/detail/detail.html**. To find book chapters, use the drop boxes at the bottom of the search page where "You may refine your search by." Select the dates and language you prefer, and the format option "Book Chapter." By making these selections and typing in "Niemann-Pick disease" (or synonyms) into the "For these words:" box, you will only receive results on chapters in books.

---

[23] In addition to LOCATORPlus, in collaboration with authors and publishers, the National Center for Biotechnology Information (NCBI) is adapting biomedical books for the Web. The books may be accessed in two ways: (1) by searching directly using any search term or phrase (in the same way as the bibliographic database PubMed), or (2) by following the links to PubMed abstracts. Each PubMed abstract has a "Books" button that displays a facsimile of the abstract in which some phrases are hypertext links. These phrases are also found in the books available at NCBI. Click on hyperlinked results in the list of books in which the phrase is found. Currently, the majority of the links are between the books and PubMed. In the future, more links will be created between the books and other types of information, such as gene and protein sequences and macromolecular structures. See **http://www.ncbi.nlm.nih.gov/entrez/query.fcgi?db=Books.**

General Home References

In addition to references for Niemann-Pick disease, you may want a general home medical guide that spans all aspects of home healthcare. The following list is a recent sample of such guides (sorted alphabetically by title; hyperlinks provide rankings, information, and reviews at Amazon.com):

- **Adams & Victor's Principles Of Neurology** by Maurice Victor, et al; Hardcover - 1692 pages; 7th edition (December 19, 2000), McGraw-Hill Professional Publishing; ISBN: 0070674973; http://www.amazon.com/exec/obidos/ASIN/0070674973/icongroupinterna

- **American Academy of Pediatrics Guide to Your Child's Symptoms : The Official, Complete Home Reference, Birth Through Adolescence** by Donald Schiff (Editor), et al; Paperback - 256 pages (January 1997), Villard Books; ISBN: 0375752579; http://www.amazon.com/exec/obidos/ASIN/0375752579/icongroupinterna

- **The Children's Hospital Guide to Your Child's Health and Development** by Alan D. Woolf (Editor), et al; Hardcover - 796 pages, 1st edition (January 15, 2001), Perseus Books; ISBN: 073820241X; http://www.amazon.com/exec/obidos/ASIN/073820241X/icongroupinterna

- **Clinical Neuroanatomy Made Ridiculously Simple (MedMaster Series, 2000 Edition)** by Stephen Goldberg; Paperback: 97 pages; 2nd edition (February 15, 2000), Medmaster; ISBN: 0940780461; http://www.amazon.com/exec/obidos/ASIN/0940780461/icongroupinterna

- **Helping Your Child in the Hospital: A Practical Guide for Parents** by Nancy Keene, Rachel Prentice; Paperback - 176 pages, 3rd edition (April 15, 2002), O'Reilly & Associates; ISBN: 0596500114; http://www.amazon.com/exec/obidos/ASIN/0596500114/icongroupinterna

- **It's Not a Tumor!: The Patient's Guide to Common Neurological Problems** by Robert Wiedemeyer; Paperback: (January 1996), Boxweed Pub; ISBN: 0964740796; http://www.amazon.com/exec/obidos/ASIN/0964740796/icongroupinterna

- **Medical Emergencies & Childhood Illnesses: Includes Your Child's Personal Health Journal (Parent Smart)** by Penny A. Shore, William Sears (Contributor); Paperback - 115 pages (February 2002), Parent Kit Corporation; ISBN: 1896833187; http://www.amazon.com/exec/obidos/ASIN/1896833187/icongroupinterna

- **Neurology for the Non-Neurologist** by William J. Weiner (Editor), Christopher G. Goetz (Editor); Paperback (May 1999), Lippincott, Williams

& Wilkins Publishers; ISBN: 0781717078;
http://www.amazon.com/exec/obidos/ASIN/0781717078/icongroupinterna

- **Taking Care of Your Child: A Parent's Guide to Complete Medical Care** by Robert H. Pantell, M.D., et al; Paperback - 524 pages, 6th edition (March 5, 2002), Perseus Press; ISBN: 0738206016;
http://www.amazon.com/exec/obidos/ASIN/0738206016/icongroupinterna

PART III. APPENDICES

ABOUT PART III

Part III is a collection of appendices on general medical topics relating to Niemann-Pick disease and related conditions.

APPENDIX A. RESEARCHING YOUR CHILD'S MEDICATIONS

Overview

There are a number of sources available on new or existing medications which could be prescribed to treat Niemann-Pick disease. While a number of hard copy or CD-Rom resources are available to parents and physicians for research purposes, a more flexible method is to use Internet-based databases. In this chapter, we will begin with a general overview of medications. We will then proceed to outline official recommendations on how you should view your child's medications. You may also want to research medications that your child is currently taking for other conditions as they may interact with medications for Niemann-Pick disease. Research can give you information on the side effects, interactions, and limitations of prescription drugs used in the treatment of Niemann-Pick disease. Broadly speaking, there are two sources of information on approved medications: public sources and private sources. We will emphasize free-to-use public sources.

Your Child's Medications: The Basics[24]

The Agency for Health Care Research and Quality has published extremely useful guidelines on the medication aspects of Niemann-Pick disease. Giving your child medication can involve many steps and decisions each day. The AHCRQ recommends that parents take part in treatment decisions. Do not be afraid to ask questions and talk about your concerns. By taking a moment to ask questions, your child may be spared from possible problems. Here are some points to cover each time a new medicine is prescribed:

---

[24] This section is adapted from AHCRQ: **http://www.ahcpr.gov/consumer/ncpiebro.htm**.

- Ask about all parts of your child's treatment, including diet changes, exercise, and medicines.
- Ask about the risks and benefits of each medicine or other treatment your child might receive.
- Ask how often you or your child's doctor will check for side effects from a given medication.

Do not hesitate to tell the doctor about preferences you have for your child's medicines. You may want your child to have a medicine with the fewest side effects, or the fewest doses to take each day. You may care most about cost. Or, you may want the medicine the doctor believes will work the best. Sharing your concerns will help the doctor select the best treatment for your child.

Do not be afraid to "bother" the doctor with your questions about medications for Niemann-Pick disease. You can also talk to a nurse or a pharmacist. They can help you better understand your child's treatment plan. Talking over your child's options with someone you trust can help you make better choices. Specifically, ask the doctor the following:

- The name of the medicine and what it is supposed to do.
- How and when to give your child the medicine, how much, and for how long.
- What food, drinks, other medicines, or activities your child should avoid while taking the medicine.
- What side effects your child may experience, and what to do if they occur.
- If there are any refills, and how often.
- About any terms or directions you do not understand.
- What to do if your child misses a dose.
- If there is written information you can take home (most pharmacies have information sheets on prescription medicines; some even offer large-print or Spanish versions).

Do not forget to tell the doctor about all the medicines your child is currently taking (not just those for Niemann-Pick disease). This includes prescription medicines and the medicines that you buy over the counter. When talking to the doctor, you may wish to prepare a list of medicines your child is currently taking including why and in what forms. Be sure to include the following information for each:

- Name of medicine
- Reason taken
- Dosage
- Time(s) of day

Also include any over-the-counter medicines, such as:
- Laxatives
- Diet pills
- Vitamins
- Cold medicine
- Aspirin or other pain, headache, or fever medicine
- Cough medicine
- Allergy relief medicine
- Antacids
- Sleeping pills
- Others (include names)

Learning More about Your Child's Medications

Because of historical investments by various organizations and the emergence of the Internet, it has become rather simple to learn about the medications the doctor has recommended for Niemann-Pick disease. One such source is the United States Pharmacopeia. In 1820, eleven physicians met in Washington, D.C. to establish the first compendium of standard drugs for the United States. They called this compendium the "U.S. Pharmacopeia (USP)." Today, the USP is a non-profit organization consisting of 800 volunteer scientists, eleven elected officials, and 400 representatives of state associations and colleges of medicine and pharmacy. The USP is located in Rockville, Maryland, and its home page is located at **www.usp.org**. The USP currently provides standards for over 3,700 medications. The resulting USP DI® Advice for the Patient® can be accessed through the National

Library of Medicine of the National Institutes of Health. The database is partially derived from lists of federally approved medications in the Food and Drug Administration's (FDA) Drug Approvals database.[25]

While the FDA database is rather large and difficult to navigate, the Phamacopeia is both user-friendly and free to use. It covers more than 9,000 prescription and over-the-counter medications. To access this database, simply type the following hyperlink into your Web browser: **http://www.nlm.nih.gov/medlineplus/druginformation.html**. To view examples of a given medication (brand names, category, description, preparation, proper use, precautions, side effects, etc.), simply follow the hyperlinks indicated within the United States Pharmacopoeia (USP). It is important to read the disclaimer by the USP (**http://www.nlm.nih.gov/medlineplus/drugdisclaimer.html**) before using the information provided.

Commercial Databases

In addition to the medications listed in the USP above, a number of commercial sites are available by subscription to physicians and their institutions. You may be able to access these sources from your local medical library or your child's doctor's office.

Reuters Health Drug Database

The Reuters Health Drug Database can be searched by keyword at the hyperlink: **http://www.reutershealth.com/frame2/drug.html**.

Mosby's GenRx

Mosby's GenRx database (also available on CD-Rom and book format) covers 45,000 drug products including generics and international brands. It provides information on prescribing and drug interactions. Information can be obtained at **http://www.genrx.com/Mosby/PhyGenRx/group.html**.

---

[25] Though cumbersome, the FDA database can be freely browsed at the following site: **www.fda.gov/cder/da/da.htm**.

Physicians Desk Reference

The Physicians Desk Reference database (also available in CD-Rom and book format) is a full-text drug database. The database is searchable by brand name, generic name or by indication. It features multiple drug interactions reports. Information can be obtained at the following hyperlink: **http://physician.pdr.net/physician/templates/en/acl/psuser_t.htm**.

Other Web Sites

A number of additional Web sites discuss drug information. As an example, you may like to look at **www.drugs.com** which reproduces the information in the Pharmacopeia as well as commercial information. You may also want to consider the Web site of the Medical Letter, Inc. which allows users to download articles on various drugs and therapeutics for a nominal fee: **http://www.medletter.com/**.

Contraindications and Interactions (Hidden Dangers)

Some of the medications mentioned in the previous discussions can be problematic for children with Niemann-Pick disease--not because they are used in the treatment process, but because of contraindications, or side effects. Medications with contraindications are those that could react with drugs used to treat Niemann-Pick disease or potentially create deleterious side effects in patients with Niemann-Pick disease. You should ask the physician about any contraindications, especially as these might apply to other medications that your child may be taking for common ailments.

Drug-drug interactions occur when two or more drugs react with each other. This drug-drug interaction may cause your child to experience an unexpected side effect. Drug interactions may make medications less effective, cause unexpected side effects, or increase the action of a particular drug. Some drug interactions can even be harmful to your child.

Be sure to read the label every time you give your child a nonprescription or prescription drug, and take the time to learn about drug interactions. These precautions may be critical to your child's health. You can reduce the risk of potentially harmful drug interactions and side effects with a little bit of knowledge and common sense.

Drug labels contain important information about ingredients, uses, warnings, and directions which you should take the time to read and understand. Labels also include warnings about possible drug interactions. Further, drug labels may change as new information becomes avaiable. This is why it's especially important to read the label every time you give your child a medication. When the doctor prescribes a new drug, discuss all over-the-counter and prescription medications, dietary supplements, vitamins, botanicals, minerals and herbals your child takes. Ask your pharmacist for the package insert for each drug prescribed. The package insert provides more information about potential drug interactions.

A Final Warning

At some point, you may hear of alternative medications from friends, relatives, or in the news media. Advertisements may suggest that certain alternative drugs can produce positive results for Niemann-Pick disease. Exercise caution--some of these drugs may have fraudulent claims, and others may actually hurt your child. The Food and Drug Administration (FDA) is the official U.S. agency charged with discovering which medications are likely to improve the health of patients with Niemann-Pick disease. The FDA warns to watch out for[26]:

- Secret formulas (real scientists share what they know)
- Amazing breakthroughs or miracle cures (real breakthroughs don't happen very often; when they do, real scientists do not call them amazing or miracles)
- Quick, painless, or guaranteed cures
- If it sounds too good to be true, it probably isn't true.

If you have any questions about any kind of medical treatment, the FDA may have an office near you. Look for their number in the blue pages of the phone book. You can also contact the FDA through its toll-free number, 1-888-INFO-FDA (1-888-463-6332), or on the World Wide Web at **www.fda.gov**.

---

[26] This section has been adapted from
http://www.fda.gov/opacom/lowlit/medfraud.html.

General References

In addition to the resources provided earlier in this chapter, the following general references describe medications (sorted alphabetically by title; hyperlinks provide rankings, information and reviews at Amazon.com):

- **Current Therapy in Neurologic Disease** by Richard T. Johnson, et al; Hardcover - 457 pages, 6th edition (January 15, 2002), Mosby-Year Book; ISBN: 0323014720;
  http://www.amazon.com/exec/obidos/ASIN/0323014720/icongroupinterna

- **Emerging Pharmacological Tools in Clinical Neurology** by MedPanel Inc. (Author); Digital - 66 pages, MarketResearch.com; ISBN: B00005RBN8; http://www.amazon.com/exec/obidos/ASIN/B00005RBN8/icongroupinterna

- **Goodman & Gilman's The Pharmacological Basis of Therapeutics by** Joel G. Hardman (Editor), Lee E. Limbird; Hardcover - 1825 pages, 10th edition (August 13, 2001), McGraw-Hill Professional Publishing; ISBN: 0071354697;
  http://www.amazon.com/exec/obidos/ASIN/0071354697/icongroupinterna

- **Neurology and General Medicine** by Michael J. Aminoff (Editor), Hardcover - 992 pages, 3rd edition (March 15, 2001), Churchill Livingstone; ISBN: 0443065713;
  http://www.amazon.com/exec/obidos/ASIN/0443065713/icongroupinterna

- **Neurology and Medicine** by Hughes Perkins; Hardcover - 415 pages, 1st edition (December 15, 1999), B. M. J. Books; ISBN: 0727912240;
  http://www.amazon.com/exec/obidos/ASIN/0727912240/icongroupinterna

- **Pharmacological Management of Neurological and Psychiatric Disorders** by S. J. Enna (Editor), et al; Hardcover - 736 pages, 1st edition, McGraw-Hill Professional Publishing; ISBN: 0070217645;
  http://www.amazon.com/exec/obidos/ASIN/0070217645/icongroupinterna

APPENDIX B. RESEARCHING NUTRITION

Overview

Since the time of Hippocrates, doctors have understood the importance of diet and nutrition to health and well-being. Since then, they have accumulated an impressive archive of studies and knowledge dedicated to this subject. Based on their experience, doctors and healthcare providers may recommend particular dietary supplements for Niemann-Pick disease. Any dietary recommendation is based on age, body mass, gender, lifestyle, eating habits, food preferences, and health condition. It is therefore likely that different patients with Niemann-Pick disease may be given different recommendations. Some recommendations may be directly related to Niemann-Pick disease, while others may be more related to general health.

In this chapter we will begin by briefly reviewing the essentials of diet and nutrition that will broadly frame more detailed discussions of Niemann-Pick disease. We will then show you how to find studies dedicated specifically to nutrition and Niemann-Pick disease.

Food and Nutrition: General Principles

What Are Essential Foods?

Food is generally viewed by official sources as consisting of six basic elements: (1) fluids, (2) carbohydrates, (3) protein, (4) fats, (5) vitamins, and (6) minerals. Consuming a combination of these elements is considered to be a healthy diet:

- **Fluids** are essential to human life as 80-percent of the body is composed of water. Water is lost via urination, sweating, diarrhea, vomiting, diuretics (drugs that increase urination), caffeine, and physical exertion.
- **Carbohydrates** are the main source for human energy (thermoregulation) and the bulk of typical diets. They are mostly classified as being either simple or complex. Simple carbohydrates include sugars which are often consumed in the form of cookies, candies, or cakes. Complex carbohydrates consist of starches and dietary fibers. Starches are consumed in the form of pastas, breads, potatoes, rice, and other foods. Soluble fibers can be eaten in the form of certain vegetables, fruits, oats, and legumes. Insoluble fibers include brown rice, whole grains, certain fruits, wheat bran and legumes.
- **Proteins** are eaten to build and repair human tissues. Some foods that are high in protein are also high in fat and calories. Food sources for protein include nuts, meat, fish, cheese, and other dairy products.
- **Fats** are consumed for both energy and the absorption of certain vitamins. There are many types of fats, with many general publications recommending the intake of unsaturated fats or those low in cholesterol.

Vitamins and minerals are fundamental to human health, growth, and, in some cases, disease prevention. Most are consumed in your child's diet (exceptions being vitamins K and D which are produced by intestinal bacteria and sunlight on the skin, respectively). Each vitamin and mineral plays a different role in health. The following outlines essential vitamins:

- **Vitamin A** is important to the health of eyes, hair, bones, and skin; sources of vitamin A include foods such as eggs, carrots, and cantaloupe.
- **Vitamin B^1**, also known as thiamine, is important for the nervous system and energy production; food sources for thiamine include meat, peas, fortified cereals, bread, and whole grains.
- **Vitamin B^2**, also known as riboflavin, is important for the nervous system and muscles, but is also involved in the release of proteins from

nutrients; food sources for riboflavin include dairy products, leafy vegetables, meat, and eggs.

- **Vitamin B^3**, also known as niacin, is important for healthy skin and helps the body use energy; food sources for niacin include peas, peanuts, fish, and whole grains
- **Vitamin B^6**, also known as pyridoxine, is important for the regulation of cells in the nervous system and is vital for blood formation; food sources for pyridoxine include bananas, whole grains, meat, and fish.
- **Vitamin B^{12}** is vital for a healthy nervous system and for the growth of red blood cells in bone marrow; food sources for vitamin B^{12} include yeast, milk, fish, eggs, and meat.
- **Vitamin C** allows the body's immune system to fight various medical conditions, strengthens body tissue, and improves the body's use of iron; food sources for vitamin C include a wide variety of fruits and vegetables.
- **Vitamin D** helps the body absorb calcium which strengthens bones and teeth; food sources for vitamin D include oily fish and dairy products.
- **Vitamin E** can help protect certain organs and tissues from various degenerative diseases; food sources for vitamin E include margarine, vegetables, eggs, and fish.
- **Vitamin K** is essential for bone formation and blood clotting; common food sources for vitamin K include leafy green vegetables.
- **Folic Acid** maintains healthy cells and blood; food sources for folic acid include nuts, fortified breads, leafy green vegetables, and whole grains.

It should be noted that one can overdose on certain vitamins which become toxic if consumed in excess (e.g. vitamin A, D, E and K).

Like vitamins, minerals are chemicals that are required by the body to remain in good health. Because the human body does not manufacture these chemicals internally, we obtain them from food and other dietary sources. The more important minerals include:

- **Calcium** is needed for healthy bones, teeth, and muscles, but also helps the nervous system function; food sources for calcium include dry beans, peas, eggs, and dairy products.
- **Chromium** is helpful in regulating sugar levels in blood; food sources for chromium include egg yolks, raw sugar, cheese, nuts, beets, whole grains, and meat.

- **Fluoride** is used by the body to help prevent tooth decay and to reinforce bone strength; sources of fluoride include drinking water and certain brands of toothpaste.
- **Iodine** helps regulate the body's use of energy by synthesizing into the hormone thyroxine; food sources include leafy green vegetables, nuts, egg yolks, and red meat.
- **Iron** helps maintain muscles and the formation of red blood cells and certain proteins; food sources for iron include meat, dairy products, eggs, and leafy green vegetables.
- **Magnesium** is important for the production of DNA, as well as for healthy teeth, bones, muscles, and nerves; food sources for magnesium include dried fruit, dark green vegetables, nuts, and seafood.
- **Phosphorous** is used by the body to work with calcium to form bones and teeth; food sources for phosphorous include eggs, meat, cereals, and dairy products.
- **Selenium** primarily helps maintain normal heart and liver functions; food sources for selenium include wholegrain cereals, fish, meat, and dairy products.
- **Zinc** helps wounds heal, the formation of sperm, and encourage rapid growth and energy; food sources include dried beans, shellfish, eggs, and nuts.

The United States government periodically publishes recommended diets and consumption levels of the various elements of food. Again, the doctor may encourage deviations from the average official recommendation based on your child's specific condition. To learn more about basic dietary guidelines, visit the Web site: **http://www.health.gov/dietaryguidelines/**. Based on these guidelines, many foods are required to list the nutrition levels on the food's packaging. Labeling Requirements are listed at the following site maintained by the Food and Drug Administration: **http://www.cfsan.fda.gov/~dms/lab-cons.html**. When interpreting these requirements, the government recommends that consumers become familiar with the following abbreviations before reading FDA literature:[27]

- **DVs (Daily Values):** A new dietary reference term that will appear on the food label. It is made up of two sets of references, DRVs and RDIs.
- **DRVs (Daily Reference Values):** A set of dietary references that applies to fat, saturated fat, cholesterol, carbohydrate, protein, fiber, sodium, and potassium.

---

[27] Adapted from the FDA: **http://www.fda.gov/fdac/special/foodlabel/dvs.html**.

- **RDIs (Reference Daily Intakes):** A set of dietary references based on the Recommended Dietary Allowances for essential vitamins and minerals and, in selected groups, protein. The name "RDI" replaces the term "U.S. RDA."
- **RDAs (Recommended Dietary Allowances):** A set of estimated nutrient allowances established by the National Academy of Sciences. It is updated periodically to reflect current scientific knowledge.

What Are Dietary Supplements?[28]

Dietary supplements are widely available through many commercial sources, including health food stores, grocery stores, pharmacies, and by mail. Dietary supplements are provided in many forms including tablets, capsules, powders, gel-tabs, extracts, and liquids. Historically in the United States, the most prevalent type of dietary supplement was a multivitamin/mineral tablet or capsule that was available in pharmacies, either by prescription or "over the counter." Supplements containing strictly herbal preparations were less widely available. Currently in the United States, a wide array of supplement products are available, including vitamin, mineral, other nutrients, and botanical supplements as well as ingredients and extracts of animal and plant origin.

The Office of Dietary Supplements (ODS) of the National Institutes of Health is the official agency of the United States which has the expressed goal of acquiring "new knowledge to help prevent, detect, diagnose, and treat disease and disability, from the rarest genetic disorder to the common cold."[29] According to the ODS, dietary supplements can have an important impact on the prevention and management of medical conditions and on the maintenance of health.[30] The ODS notes that considerable research on the effects of dietary supplements has been conducted in Asia and Europe where the use of plant products, in particular, has a long tradition. However, the

---

[28] This discussion has been adapted from the NIH: http://ods.od.nih.gov/whatare/whatare.html.

[29] Contact: The Office of Dietary Supplements, National Institutes of Health, Building 31, Room 1B29, 31 Center Drive, MSC 2086, Bethesda, Maryland 20892-2086, Tel: (301) 435-2920, Fax: (301) 480-1845, E-mail: **ods@nih.gov**.

[30] Adapted from **http://ods.od.nih.gov/about/about.html**. The Dietary Supplement Health and Education Act defines dietary supplements as "a product (other than tobacco) intended to supplement the diet that bears or contains one or more of the following dietary ingredients: a vitamin, mineral, amino acid, herb or other botanical; or a dietary substance for use to supplement the diet by increasing the total dietary intake; or a concentrate, metabolite, constituent, extract, or combination of any ingredient described above; and intended for ingestion in the form of a capsule, powder, softgel, or gelcap, and not represented as a conventional food or as a sole item of a meal or the diet."

overwhelming majority of supplements have not been studied scientifically. To explore the role of dietary supplements in the improvement of health care, the ODS plans, organizes, and supports conferences, workshops, and symposia on scientific topics related to dietary supplements. The ODS often works in conjunction with other NIH Institutes and Centers, other government agencies, professional organizations, and public advocacy groups.

To learn more about official information on dietary supplements, visit the ODS site at **http://ods.od.nih.gov/whatare/whatare.html**. Or contact:

> The Office of Dietary Supplements
> National Institutes of Health
> Building 31, Room 1B29
> 31 Center Drive, MSC 2086
> Bethesda, Maryland 20892-2086
> Tel: (301) 435-2920
> Fax: (301) 480-1845
> E-mail: ods@nih.gov

Finding Studies on Niemann-Pick Disease

The NIH maintains an office dedicated to nutrition and diet. The National Institutes of Health's Office of Dietary Supplements (ODS) offers a searchable bibliographic database called the IBIDS (International Bibliographic Information on Dietary Supplements). The IBIDS contains over 460,000 scientific citations and summaries about dietary supplements and nutrition as well as references to published international, scientific literature on dietary supplements such as vitamins, minerals, and botanicals.[31] IBIDS is available to the public free of charge through the ODS Internet page: **http://ods.od.nih.gov/databases/ibids.html**.

After entering the search area, you have three choices: (1) IBIDS Consumer Database, (2) Full IBIDS Database, or (3) Peer Reviewed Citations Only. We recommend that you start with the Consumer Database. While you may not find references for the topics that are of most interest to you, check back periodically as this database is frequently updated. More studies can be

---

[31] Adapted from http://ods.od.nih.gov. IBIDS is produced by the Office of Dietary Supplements (ODS) at the National Institutes of Health to assist the public, healthcare providers, educators, and researchers in locating credible, scientific information on dietary supplements. IBIDS was developed and will be maintained through an interagency partnership with the Food and Nutrition Information Center of the National Agricultural Library, U.S. Department of Agriculture.

found by searching the Full IBIDS Database. Healthcare professionals and researchers generally use the third option, which lists peer-reviewed citations. In all cases, we suggest that you take advantage of the "Advanced Search" option that allows you to retrieve up to 100 fully explained references in a comprehensive format. Type "Niemann-Pick disease" (or synonyms) into the search box. To narrow the search, you can also select the "Title" field.

The following information is typical of that found when using the "Full IBIDS Database" when searching using "Niemann-Pick disease" (or a synonym):

- **Cell autonomous apoptosis defects in acid sphingomyelinase knockout fibroblasts.**
  Author(s): Laboratory of Signal Transduction and Department of Radiation Oncology, Memorial Sloan-Kettering Cancer Center, New York, New York 10021, USA.
  Source: Lozano, J Menendez, S Morales, A Ehleiter, D Liao, W C Wagman, R Haimovitz Friedman, A Fuks, Z Kolesnick, R J-Biol-Chem. 2001 January 5; 276(1): 442-8 0021-9258

- **Complete removal of sphingolipids from the plasma membrane disrupts cell to substratum adhesion of mouse melanoma cells.**
  Author(s): Laboratory for Cellular Glycobiology, Frontier Research Program, Institute of Physical and Chemical Research (RIKEN), 2-1, Hirosawa, Wako-shi, Saitama 351-01, Japan.
  Source: Hidari KIPJ Ichikawa, S Fujita, T Sakiyama, H Hirabayashi, Y J-Biol-Chem. 1996 June 14; 271(24): 14636-41 0021-9258

- **Cyclodextrins in the treatment of a mouse model of Niemann-Pick C disease.**
  Author(s): Steele Memorial Children's Research Center, Department of Pediatrics, The University of Arizona College of Medicine, Tucson 85724, USA.
  Source: Camargo, F Erickson, R P Garver, W S Hossain, G S Carbone, P N Heidenreich, R A Blanchard, J Life-Sci. 2001 November 30; 70(2): 131-42 0024-3205

- **Degradation of fluorescent and radiolabelled sphingomyelins in intact cells by a non-lysosomal pathway.**
  Author(s): Laboratoire de Biochimie, CJF INSERM 9206, Institut Louis Bugnard, C.H.U. Rangueil, Toulouse, France.
  Source: Levade, T Vidal, F Vermeersch, S Andrieu, N Gatt, S Salvayre, R Biochim-Biophys-Acta. 1995 October 5; 1258(3): 277-87 0006-3002

- **Distribution of acid sphingomyelinase in human various body fluids.**
  Author(s): Department of Pediatrics, University School of Medicine, Akita, Japan. tomy@med.akita-u.ac.jp
  Source: Takahashi, I Takahashi, T Abe, T Watanabe, W Takada, G Tohoku-J-Exp-Med. 2000 September; 192(1): 61-6 0040-8727

- **Effects of dietary cholesterol restriction in a feline model of Niemann-Pick type C disease.**
  Author(s): Department of Pathology, Colorado State University, Fort Collins 80523, USA.
  Source: Somers, K L Brown, D E Fulton, R Schultheiss, P C HaMarch, D Smith, M O Allison, R Connally, H E Just, C Mitchell, T W Wenger, D A Thrall, M A J-Inherit-Metab-Dis. 2001 August; 24(4): 427-36 0141-8955

- **Expression of Niemann-Pick type C transcript in rodent cerebellum in vivo and in vitro.**
  Author(s): Department of Physiology, University of Arizona College of Medicine, Tucson, AZ 85724-5051, USA. tfalk@u.arizona.edu
  Source: Falk, T Garver, W S Erickson, R P Wilson, J M Yool, A J Brain-Res. 1999 August 21; 839(1): 49-57 0006-8993

- **Incorporation of polyunsaturated fatty acids into bis(monoacylglycero)phosphate and other lipids of macrophages and of fibroblasts from control and Niemann-Pick patients.**
  Source: Huterer, S Wherrett, J R Biochim-Biophys-Acta. 1986 April 15; 876(2): 318-26 0006-3002

- **Involvement of the acid sphingomyelinase pathway in uva-induced apoptosis.**
  Author(s): Hormel Institute, University of Minnesota, Austin, Minnesota 55912, USA.
  Source: Zhang, Y Mattjus, P Schmid, P C Dong, Z Zhong, S Ma, W Y Brown, R E Bode, A M Schmid, H H Dong, Z J-Biol-Chem. 2001 April 13; 276(15): 11775-82 0021-9258

- **Late endosomal membranes rich in lysobisphosphatidic acid regulate cholesterol transport.**
  Author(s): Department of Biochemistry, University of Geneva, Switzerland.
  Source: Kobayashi, T Beuchat, M H Lindsay, M Frias, S Palmiter, R D Sakuraba, H Parton, R G Gruenberg, J Nat-Cell-Biol. 1999 June; 1(2): 113-8 1465-7392

- **L-selectin stimulates the neutral sphingomyelinase and induces release of ceramide.**
  Author(s): Department of Neonatology, University of Tuebingen, Ruemelinstrasse 23, Tuebingen, 72070, Germany.

Source: Brenner, B Grassme, H U Muller, C Lang, F Speer, C P Gulbins, E Exp-Cell-Res. 1998 August 25; 243(1): 123-8 0014-4827

- **Macrophage-released proteoglycans enhance LDL aggregation: studies in aorta from apolipoprotein E-deficient mice.**
  Author(s): The Lipid Research Laboratory, The Bruce Rappaport Faculty of Medicine, Technion, The Rappaport Family Institute for Research in the Medical Sciences and Rambam Medical Center, Haifa, Israel.
  Source: Maor, I Hayek, T Hirsh, M Iancu, T C Aviram, M Atherosclerosis. 2000 May; 150(1): 91-101 0021-9150

- **Magnetic resonance spectroscopy in Niemann-Pick disease type C: correlation with diagnosis and clinical response to cholestyramine and lovastatin.**
  Author(s): Department of Neurology/NeuroSurgery, McGill University, Montreal, Canada.
  Source: Sylvain, M Arnold, D L Scriver, C R Schreiber, R Shevell, M I Pediatr-Neurol. 1994 May; 10(3): 228-32 0887-8994

- **Myocardial changes in newborn piglets fed sow milk or milk replacer diets containing different levels of erucic acid.**
  Author(s): Animal Research Center, Agriculture Canada, Ottawa, Ontario.
  Source: Kramer, J K Farnworth, E R Johnston, K M Wolynetz, M S Modler, H W Sauer, F D Lipids. 1990 November; 25(11): 729-37 0024-4201

- **Niemann-Pick disease type C and defective peroxisomal beta-oxidation of branched-chain substrates.**
  Author(s): Institute of Child Health, London, UK.
  Source: Sequeira, J S Vellodi, A Vanier, M T Clayton, P T J-Inherit-Metab-Dis. 1998 April; 21(2): 149-54 0141-8955

- **Niemann-Pick disease types C and D.**
  Author(s): Developmental and Metabolic Neurology Branch, National Institute of Neurological and Communicative Disorders and Stroke, Bethesda, Maryland.
  Source: Brady, R O Filling Katz, M R Barton, N W Pentchev, P G Neurol-Clin. 1989 February; 7(1): 75-88 0733-8619

- **Photosensitization of cultured cells and viruses by pyrene lipids.**
  Author(s): Department of Membrane Biochemistry, Hebrew University, Hadassah School of Medicine, Jerusalem, Israel.
  Source: Gatt, S Dinur, T Abou Rabia, S Kotler, M Fibach, E Indian-J-Biochem-Biophys. 1990 December; 27(6): 359-62 0301-1208

- **Reduced cholesterol accumulation and improved deficient peroxisomal functions in a murine model of Niemann-Pick type C disease upon treatment with peroxisomal proliferators.**
  Author(s): Department of Biochemistry, Stockholm University, Sweden. fia@biokemi.su.se
  Source: Schedin, S Pentchev, P Dallner, G Biochem-Pharmacol. 1998 November 1; 56(9): 1195-9 0006-2952

- **Sphingomyelin metabolism in rat liver after chronic dietary replacement of choline by N-aminodeanol.**
  Author(s): Department of Biochemistry, Emory University School of Medicine, Atlanta, GA 30322-3050, USA.
  Source: Nikolova Karakashian, M N Russell, R W Booth, R A Jenden, D J Merrill, A H J-Lipid-Res. 1997 September; 38(9): 1764-70 0022-2275

- **The effect of cholesterol-lowering agents on hepatic and plasma cholesterol in Niemann-Pick disease type C.**
  Author(s): Developmental and Metabolic Neurology Branch, National Institute of Neurological Disorders and Stroke, National Institutes of Health, Bethesda, MD 20892.
  Source: Patterson, M C Di Bisceglie, A M Higgins, J J Abel, R B Schiffmann, R Parker, C C Argoff, C E Grewal, R P Yu, K Pentchev, P G et al. Neurology. 1993 January; 43(1): 61-4 0028-3878

Federal Resources on Nutrition

In addition to the IBIDS, the United States Department of Health and Human Services (HHS) and the United States Department of Agriculture (USDA) provide many sources of information on general nutrition and health. Recommended resources include:

- healthfinder®, HHS's gateway to health information, including diet and nutrition:
  http://www.healthfinder.gov/scripts/SearchContext.asp?topic=238&page=0

- The United States Department of Agriculture's Web site dedicated to nutrition information: **www.nutrition.gov**

- The Food and Drug Administration's Web site for federal food safety information: **www.foodsafety.gov**

- The National Action Plan on Overweight and Obesity sponsored by the United States Surgeon General:
  http://www.surgeongeneral.gov/topics/obesity/

- The Center for Food Safety and Applied Nutrition has an Internet site sponsored by the Food and Drug Administration and the Department of Health and Human Services: **http://vm.cfsan.fda.gov/**
- Center for Nutrition Policy and Promotion sponsored by the United States Department of Agriculture: **http://www.usda.gov/cnpp/**
- Food and Nutrition Information Center, National Agricultural Library sponsored by the United States Department of Agriculture: **http://www.nal.usda.gov/fnic/**
- Food and Nutrition Service sponsored by the United States Department of Agriculture: **http://www.fns.usda.gov/fns/**

Additional Web Resources

A number of additional Web sites offer encyclopedic information covering food and nutrition. The following is a representative sample:

- AOL: **http://search.aol.com/cat.adp?id=174&layer=&from=subcats**
- Family Village: **http://www.familyvillage.wisc.edu/med_nutrition.html**
- Google: **http://directory.google.com/Top/Health/Nutrition/**
- Healthnotes: **http://www.thedacare.org/healthnotes/**
- Open Directory Project: **http://dmoz.org/Health/Nutrition/**
- Yahoo.com: **http://dir.yahoo.com/Health/Nutrition/**
- WebMD®Health: **http://my.webmd.com/nutrition**
- WholeHealthMD.com: **http://www.wholehealthmd.com/reflib/0,1529,,00.html**

APPENDIX C. FINDING MEDICAL LIBRARIES

Overview

At a medical library you can find medical texts and reference books, consumer health publications, specialty newspapers and magazines, as well as medical journals. In this Appendix, we show you how to quickly find a medical library in your area.

Preparation

Before going to the library, highlight the references mentioned in this sourcebook that you find interesting. Focus on those items that are not available via the Internet, and ask the reference librarian for help with your search. He or she may know of additional resources that could be helpful to you. Most importantly, your local public library and medical libraries have Interlibrary Loan programs with the National Library of Medicine (NLM), one of the largest medical collections in the world. According to the NLM, most of the literature in the general and historical collections of the National Library of Medicine is available on interlibrary loan to any library. NLM's interlibrary loan services are only available to libraries. If you would like to access NLM medical literature, then visit a library in your area that can request the publications for you.[32]

---

[32] Adapted from the NLM: http://www.nlm.nih.gov/psd/cas/interlibrary.html.

Finding a Local Medical Library

The quickest method to locate medical libraries is to use the Internet-based directory published by the National Network of Libraries of Medicine (NN/LM). This network includes 4626 members and affiliates that provide many services to librarians, health professionals, and the public. To find a library in your area, simply visit **http://nnlm.gov/members/adv.html** or call 1-800-338-7657.

Medical Libraries Open to the Public

In addition to the NN/LM, the National Library of Medicine (NLM) lists a number of libraries that are generally open to the public and have reference facilities. The following is the NLM's list plus hyperlinks to each library Web site. These Web pages can provide information on hours of operation and other restrictions. The list below is a small sample of libraries recommended by the National Library of Medicine (sorted alphabetically by name of the U.S. state or Canadian province where the library is located):[33]

- **Alabama:** Health InfoNet of Jefferson County (Jefferson County Library Cooperative, Lister Hill Library of the Health Sciences), **http://www.uab.edu/infonet/**

- **Alabama:** Richard M. Scrushy Library (American Sports Medicine Institute), **http://www.asmi.org/LIBRARY.HTM**

- **Arizona:** Samaritan Regional Medical Center: The Learning Center (Samaritan Health System, Phoenix, Arizona), **http://www.samaritan.edu/library/bannerlibs.htm**

- **California:** Kris Kelly Health Information Center (St. Joseph Health System), **http://www.humboldt1.com/~kkhic/index.html**

- **California:** Community Health Library of Los Gatos (Community Health Library of Los Gatos), **http://www.healthlib.org/orgresources.html**

- **California:** Consumer Health Program and Services (CHIPS) (County of Los Angeles Public Library, Los Angeles County Harbor-UCLA Medical Center Library) - Carson, CA, **http://www.colapublib.org/services/chips.html**

- **California:** Gateway Health Library (Sutter Gould Medical Foundation)

- **California:** Health Library (Stanford University Medical Center), **http://www-med.stanford.edu/healthlibrary/**

---

[33] Abstracted from **http://www.nlm.nih.gov/medlineplus/libraries.html**

- **California:** Patient Education Resource Center - Health Information and Resources (University of California, San Francisco), **http://sfghdean.ucsf.edu/barnett/PERC/default.asp**
- **California:** Redwood Health Library (Petaluma Health Care District), **http://www.phcd.org/rdwdlib.html**
- **California:** San José PlaneTree Health Library, **http://planetreesanjose.org/**
- **California:** Sutter Resource Library (Sutter Hospitals Foundation), **http://go.sutterhealth.org/comm/resc-library/sac-resources.html**
- **California:** University of California, Davis. Health Sciences Libraries
- **California:** ValleyCare Health Library & Ryan Comer Cancer Resource Center (ValleyCare Health System), **http://www.valleycare.com/library.html**
- **California:** Washington Community Health Resource Library (Washington Community Health Resource Library), **http://www.healthlibrary.org/**
- **Colorado:** William V. Gervasini Memorial Library (Exempla Healthcare), **http://www.exempla.org/conslib.htm**
- **Connecticut:** Hartford Hospital Health Science Libraries (Hartford Hospital), **http://www.harthosp.org/library/**
- **Connecticut:** Healthnet: Connecticut Consumer Health Information Center (University of Connecticut Health Center, Lyman Maynard Stowe Library), **http://library.uchc.edu/departm/hnet/**
- **Connecticut:** Waterbury Hospital Health Center Library (Waterbury Hospital), **http://www.waterburyhospital.com/library/consumer.shtml**
- **Delaware:** Consumer Health Library (Christiana Care Health System, Eugene du Pont Preventive Medicine & Rehabilitation Institute), **http://www.christianacare.org/health_guide/health_guide_pmri_health_info.cfm**
- **Delaware:** Lewis B. Flinn Library (Delaware Academy of Medicine), **http://www.delamed.org/chls.html**
- **Georgia:** Family Resource Library (Medical College of Georgia), **http://cmc.mcg.edu/kids_families/fam_resources/fam_res_lib/frl.htm**
- **Georgia:** Health Resource Center (Medical Center of Central Georgia), **http://www.mccg.org/hrc/hrchome.asp**
- **Hawaii:** Hawaii Medical Library: Consumer Health Information Service (Hawaii Medical Library), **http://hml.org/CHIS/**

- **Idaho:** DeArmond Consumer Health Library (Kootenai Medical Center), http://www.nicon.org/DeArmond/index.htm
- **Illinois:** Health Learning Center of Northwestern Memorial Hospital (Northwestern Memorial Hospital, Health Learning Center), http://www.nmh.org/health_info/hlc.html
- **Illinois:** Medical Library (OSF Saint Francis Medical Center), http://www.osfsaintfrancis.org/general/library/
- **Kentucky:** Medical Library - Services for Patients, Families, Students & the Public (Central Baptist Hospital), http://www.centralbap.com/education/community/library.htm
- **Kentucky:** University of Kentucky - Health Information Library (University of Kentucky, Chandler Medical Center, Health Information Library), http://www.mc.uky.edu/PatientEd/
- **Louisiana:** Alton Ochsner Medical Foundation Library (Alton Ochsner Medical Foundation), http://www.ochsner.org/library/
- **Louisiana:** Louisiana State University Health Sciences Center Medical Library-Shreveport, http://lib-sh.lsuhsc.edu/
- **Maine:** Franklin Memorial Hospital Medical Library (Franklin Memorial Hospital), http://www.fchn.org/fmh/lib.htm
- **Maine:** Gerrish-True Health Sciences Library (Central Maine Medical Center), http://www.cmmc.org/library/library.html
- **Maine:** Hadley Parrot Health Science Library (Eastern Maine Healthcare), http://www.emh.org/hll/hpl/guide.htm
- **Maine:** Maine Medical Center Library (Maine Medical Center), http://www.mmc.org/library/
- **Maine:** Parkview Hospital, http://www.parkviewhospital.org/communit.htm#Library
- **Maine:** Southern Maine Medical Center Health Sciences Library (Southern Maine Medical Center), http://www.smmc.org/services/service.php3?choice=10
- **Maine:** Stephens Memorial Hospital Health Information Library (Western Maine Health), http://www.wmhcc.com/hil_frame.html
- **Manitoba, Canada:** Consumer & Patient Health Information Service (University of Manitoba Libraries), http://www.umanitoba.ca/libraries/units/health/reference/chis.html
- **Manitoba, Canada:** J.W. Crane Memorial Library (Deer Lodge Centre), http://www.deerlodge.mb.ca/library/libraryservices.shtml

- **Maryland:** Health Information Center at the Wheaton Regional Library (Montgomery County, Md., Dept. of Public Libraries, Wheaton Regional Library), **http://www.mont.lib.md.us/healthinfo/hic.asp**

- **Massachusetts:** Baystate Medical Center Library (Baystate Health System), **http://www.baystatehealth.com/1024/**

- **Massachusetts:** Boston University Medical Center Alumni Medical Library (Boston University Medical Center), **http://med-libwww.bu.edu/library/lib.html**

- **Massachusetts:** Lowell General Hospital Health Sciences Library (Lowell General Hospital), **http://www.lowellgeneral.org/library/HomePageLinks/WWW.htm**

- **Massachusetts:** Paul E. Woodard Health Sciences Library (New England Baptist Hospital), **http://www.nebh.org/health_lib.asp**

- **Massachusetts:** St. Luke's Hospital Health Sciences Library (St. Luke's Hospital), **http://www.southcoast.org/library/**

- **Massachusetts:** Treadwell Library Consumer Health Reference Center (Massachusetts General Hospital), **http://www.mgh.harvard.edu/library/chrcindex.html**

- **Massachusetts:** UMass HealthNet (University of Massachusetts Medical School), **http://healthnet.umassmed.edu/**

- **Michigan:** Botsford General Hospital Library - Consumer Health (Botsford General Hospital, Library & Internet Services), **http://www.botsfordlibrary.org/consumer.htm**

- **Michigan:** Helen DeRoy Medical Library (Providence Hospital and Medical Centers), **http://www.providence-hospital.org/library/**

- **Michigan:** Marquette General Hospital - Consumer Health Library (Marquette General Hospital, Health Information Center), **http://www.mgh.org/center.html**

- **Michigan:** Patient Education Resouce Center - University of Michigan Cancer Center (University of Michigan Comprehensive Cancer Center), **http://www.cancer.med.umich.edu/learn/leares.htm**

- **Michigan:** Sladen Library & Center for Health Information Resources - Consumer Health Information, **http://www.sladen.hfhs.org/library/consumer/index.html**

- **Montana:** Center for Health Information (St. Patrick Hospital and Health Sciences Center), **http://www.saintpatrick.org/chi/librarydetail.php3?ID=41**

- **National:** Consumer Health Library Directory (Medical Library Association, Consumer and Patient Health Information Section), **http://caphis.mlanet.org/directory/index.html**
- **National:** National Network of Libraries of Medicine (National Library of Medicine) - provides library services for health professionals in the United States who do not have access to a medical library, **http://nnlm.gov/**
- **National:** NN/LM List of Libraries Serving the Public (National Network of Libraries of Medicine), **http://nnlm.gov/members/**
- **Nevada:** Health Science Library, West Charleston Library (Las Vegas Clark County Library District), **http://www.lvccld.org/special_collections/medical/index.htm**
- **New Hampshire:** Dartmouth Biomedical Libraries (Dartmouth College Library), **http://www.dartmouth.edu/~biomed/resources.htmld/conshealth.htmld/**
- **New Jersey:** Consumer Health Library (Rahway Hospital), **http://www.rahwayhospital.com/library.htm**
- **New Jersey:** Dr. Walter Phillips Health Sciences Library (Englewood Hospital and Medical Center), **http://www.englewoodhospital.com/links/index.htm**
- **New Jersey:** Meland Foundation (Englewood Hospital and Medical Center), **http://www.geocities.com/ResearchTriangle/9360/**
- **New York:** Choices in Health Information (New York Public Library) - NLM Consumer Pilot Project participant, **http://www.nypl.org/branch/health/links.html**
- **New York:** Health Information Center (Upstate Medical University, State University of New York), **http://www.upstate.edu/library/hic/**
- **New York:** Health Sciences Library (Long Island Jewish Medical Center), **http://www.lij.edu/library/library.html**
- **New York:** ViaHealth Medical Library (Rochester General Hospital), **http://www.nyam.org/library/**
- **Ohio:** Consumer Health Library (Akron General Medical Center, Medical & Consumer Health Library), **http://www.akrongeneral.org/hwlibrary.htm**
- **Oklahoma:** Saint Francis Health System Patient/Family Resource Center (Saint Francis Health System), **http://www.sfh-tulsa.com/patientfamilycenter/default.asp**

- **Oregon:** Planetree Health Resource Center (Mid-Columbia Medical Center), **http://www.mcmc.net/phrc/**
- **Pennsylvania:** Community Health Information Library (Milton S. Hershey Medical Center), **http://www.hmc.psu.edu/commhealth/**
- **Pennsylvania:** Community Health Resource Library (Geisinger Medical Center), **http://www.geisinger.edu/education/commlib.shtml**
- **Pennsylvania:** HealthInfo Library (Moses Taylor Hospital), **http://www.mth.org/healthwellness.html**
- **Pennsylvania:** Hopwood Library (University of Pittsburgh, Health Sciences Library System), **http://www.hsls.pitt.edu/chi/hhrcinfo.html**
- **Pennsylvania:** Koop Community Health Information Center (College of Physicians of Philadelphia), **http://www.collphyphil.org/kooppg1.shtml**
- **Pennsylvania:** Learning Resources Center - Medical Library (Susquehanna Health System), **http://www.shscares.org/services/lrc/index.asp**
- **Pennsylvania:** Medical Library (UPMC Health System), **http://www.upmc.edu/passavant/library.htm**
- **Quebec, Canada:** Medical Library (Montreal General Hospital), **http://ww2.mcgill.ca/mghlib/**
- **South Dakota:** Rapid City Regional Hospital - Health Information Center (Rapid City Regional Hospital, Health Information Center), **http://www.rcrh.org/education/LibraryResourcesConsumers.htm**
- **Texas:** Houston HealthWays (Houston Academy of Medicine-Texas Medical Center Library), **http://hhw.library.tmc.edu/**
- **Texas:** Matustik Family Resource Center (Cook Children's Health Care System), **http://www.cookchildrens.com/Matustik_Library.html**
- **Washington:** Community Health Library (Kittitas Valley Community Hospital), **http://www.kvch.com/**
- **Washington:** Southwest Washington Medical Center Library (Southwest Washington Medical Center), **http://www.swmedctr.com/Home/**

Appendix D. Your Child's Rights and Insurance

Overview

Parents face a series of issues related more to the healthcare industry than to their children's medical conditions. This appendix covers two important topics in this regard: your responsibilities and your child's rights as a patient, and how to get the most out of your child's medical insurance plan.

Your Child's Rights as a Patient

The President's Advisory Commission on Consumer Protection and Quality in the Healthcare Industry has created the following summary of your child's rights as a patient.[34]

Information Disclosure

Consumers have the right to receive accurate, easily understood information. Some consumers require assistance in making informed decisions about health plans, health professionals, and healthcare facilities. Such information includes:

- *Health plans.* Covered benefits, cost-sharing, and procedures for resolving complaints, licensure, certification, and accreditation status, comparable measures of quality and consumer satisfaction, provider network composition, the procedures that govern access to specialists and emergency services, and care management information.

---

[34] Adapted from Consumer Bill of Rights and Responsibilities:
http://www.hcqualitycommission.gov/press/cbor.html#head1.

- *Health professionals.* Education, board certification, and recertification, years of practice, experience performing certain procedures, and comparable measures of quality and consumer satisfaction.
- *Healthcare facilities.* Experience in performing certain procedures and services, accreditation status, comparable measures of quality, worker, and consumer satisfaction, and procedures for resolving complaints.
- *Consumer assistance programs.* Programs must be carefully structured to promote consumer confidence and to work cooperatively with health plans, providers, payers, and regulators. Desirable characteristics of such programs are sponsorship that ensures accountability to the interests of consumers and stable, adequate funding.

Choice of Providers and Plans

Consumers have the right to a choice of healthcare providers that is sufficient to ensure access to appropriate high-quality healthcare. To ensure such choice, the Commission recommends the following:

- *Provider network adequacy.* All health plan networks should provide access to sufficient numbers and types of providers to assure that all covered services will be accessible without unreasonable delay -- including access to emergency services 24 hours a day and 7 days a week. If a health plan has an insufficient number or type of providers to provide a covered benefit with the appropriate degree of specialization, the plan should ensure that the consumer obtains the benefit outside the network at no greater cost than if the benefit were obtained from participating providers.
- *Access to specialists.* Consumers with complex or serious medical conditions who require frequent specialty care should have direct access to a qualified specialist of their choice within a plan's network of providers. Authorizations, when required, should be for an adequate number of direct access visits under an approved treatment plan.
- *Transitional care.* Consumers who are undergoing a course of treatment for a chronic or disabling condition at the time they involuntarily change health plans or at a time when a provider is terminated by a plan for other than cause should be able to continue seeing their current specialty providers for up to 90 days to allow for transition of care.
- *Choice of health plans.* Public and private group purchasers should, wherever feasible, offer consumers a choice of high-quality health insurance plans.

Access to Emergency Services

Consumers have the right to access emergency healthcare services when and where the need arises. Health plans should provide payment when a consumer presents to an emergency department with acute symptoms of sufficient severity--including severe pain--such that a "prudent layperson" could reasonably expect the absence of medical attention to result in placing that consumer's health in serious jeopardy, serious impairment to bodily functions, or serious dysfunction of any bodily organ or part.

Participation in Treatment Decisions

Consumers have the right and responsibility to fully participate in all decisions related to their healthcare. Consumers who are unable to fully participate in treatment decisions have the right to be represented by parents, guardians, family members, or other conservators. Physicians and other health professionals should:

- Provide parents with sufficient information and opportunity to decide among treatment options consistent with the informed consent process.

- Discuss all treatment options with a parent in a culturally competent manner, including the option of no treatment at all.

- Ensure that persons with disabilities have effective communications with members of the health system in making such decisions.

- Discuss all current treatments a consumer may be undergoing.

- Discuss all risks, benefits, and consequences to treatment or nontreatment.

- Give parents the opportunity to refuse treatment for their children and to express preferences about future treatment decisions.

- Discuss the use of advance directives -- both living wills and durable powers of attorney for healthcare -- with parents.

- Abide by the decisions made by parents consistent with the informed consent process.

Health plans, health providers, and healthcare facilities should:

- Disclose to consumers factors -- such as methods of compensation, ownership of or interest in healthcare facilities, or matters of conscience -- that could influence advice or treatment decisions.

- Assure that provider contracts do not contain any so-called "gag clauses" or other contractual mechanisms that restrict healthcare providers' ability to communicate with and advise parents about medically necessary treatment options for their children.

- Be prohibited from penalizing or seeking retribution against healthcare professionals or other health workers for advocating on behalf of their patients.

Respect and Nondiscrimination

Consumers have the right to considerate, respectful care from all members of the healthcare industry at all times and under all circumstances. An environment of mutual respect is essential to maintain a quality healthcare system. To assure that right, the Commission recommends the following:

- Consumers must not be discriminated against in the delivery of healthcare services consistent with the benefits covered in their policy, or as required by law, based on race, ethnicity, national origin, religion, sex, age, mental or physical disability, sexual orientation, genetic information, or source of payment.

- Consumers eligible for coverage under the terms and conditions of a health plan or program, or as required by law, must not be discriminated against in marketing and enrollment practices based on race, ethnicity, national origin, religion, sex, age, mental or physical disability, sexual orientation, genetic information, or source of payment.

Confidentiality of Health Information

Consumers have the right to communicate with healthcare providers in confidence and to have the confidentiality of their individually identifiable healthcare information protected. Consumers also have the right to review and copy their own medical records and request amendments to their records.

Complaints and Appeals

Consumers have the right to a fair and efficient process for resolving differences with their health plans, healthcare providers, and the institutions that serve them, including a rigorous system of internal review and an independent system of external review. A free copy of the Patient's Bill of Rights is available from the American Hospital Association.[35]

Parent Responsibilities

To underscore the importance of finance in modern healthcare as well as your responsibility for the financial aspects of your child's care, the President's Advisory Commission on Consumer Protection and Quality in the Healthcare Industry has proposed that parents understand the following "Consumer Responsibilities."[36] In a healthcare system that protects consumers' rights, it is reasonable to expect and encourage consumers to assume certain responsibilities. Greater involvement by parents in their children's care increases the likelihood of achieving the best outcome and helps support a quality-oriented, cost-conscious environment. Such responsibilities include:

- Take responsibility for maximizing your child's healthy habits.
- Work collaboratively with healthcare providers in developing and carrying out your child's agreed-upon treatment plans.
- Disclose relevant information and clearly communicate wants and needs.
- Use the insurance company's internal complaint and appeal processes to address your concerns.
- Recognize the reality of risks, the limits of the medical science, and the human fallibility of the healthcare professional.
- Be aware of a healthcare provider's obligation to be reasonably efficient and equitable in providing care to the community.
- Become knowledgeable about health plan coverage and options (when available) including all covered benefits, limitations, and exclusions, rules regarding use of network providers, coverage and referral rules,

---

[35] To order your free copy of the Patient's Bill of Rights, telephone 312-422-3000 or visit the American Hospital Association's Web site: http://www.aha.org. Click on "Resource Center," go to "Search" at bottom of page, and then type in "Patient's Bill of Rights." The Patient's Bill of Rights is also available from Fax on Demand, at 312-422-2020, document number 471124.

[36] Adapted from http://www.hcqualitycommission.gov/press/cbor.html#head1.

appropriate processes to secure additional information, and the process to appeal coverage decisions.

- Make a good-faith effort to meet financial obligations.
- Abide by administrative and operational procedures of health plans, healthcare providers, and Government health benefit programs.

Choosing an Insurance Plan

There are a number of official government agencies that help consumers understand their healthcare insurance choices.[37] The U.S. Department of Labor, in particular, recommends ten ways to make your health benefits choices work best for your family.[38]

1. Your options are important. There are many different types of health benefit plans. Find out which one your employer offers, then check out the plan, or plans, offered. Your employer's human resource office, the health plan administrator, or your union can provide information to help you match your family's needs and preferences with the available plans. The more information you have, the better your healthcare decisions will be.

2. Reviewing the benefits available. Do the plans offered cover preventive care, well-baby care, vision or dental care? Are there deductibles? Answers to these questions can help determine the out-of-pocket expenses you may face. Cheapest may not always be best. Your goal is high quality health benefits.

3. Look for quality. The quality of healthcare services varies, but quality can be measured. You should consider the quality of healthcare in deciding among the healthcare plans or options available to your family. Not all health plans, doctors, hospitals and other providers give the highest quality care. Fortunately, there is quality information you can use right now to help you compare your healthcare choices. Find out how you can measure quality. Consult the U.S. Department of Health and Human Services publication "Your Guide to Choosing Quality Health Care" on the Internet at **www.ahcpr.gov/consumer**.

---

[37] More information about quality across programs is provided at the following AHRQ Web site:
http://www.ahrq.gov/consumer/qntascii/qnthplan.htm.
[38] Adapted from the Department of Labor:
http://www.dol.gov/dol/pwba/public/pubs/health/top10-text.html.

4. Your plan's summary plan description (SPD) provides a wealth of information. Your health plan administrator can provide you with a copy of your plan's SPD. It outlines your family's benefits and your legal rights under the Employee Retirement Income Security Act (ERISA), the federal law that protects your family's health benefits. It should contain information about the coverage of dependents, what services will require a co-pay, and the circumstances under which your employer can change or terminate a health benefits plan. Save the SPD and all other health plan brochures and documents, along with memos or correspondence from your employer relating to health benefits.

5. Assess your benefit coverage as your family status changes. Marriage, divorce, childbirth or adoption, and the death of a spouse are all life events that may signal a need to change your health benefits. You, your spouse and dependent children may be eligible for a special enrollment period under provisions of the Health Insurance Portability and Accountability Act (HIPAA). Even without life-changing events, the information provided by your employer should tell you how you can change benefits or switch plans, if more than one plan is offered. If your spouse's employer also offers a health benefits package, consider coordinating both plans for maximum coverage.

6. Changing jobs and other life events can affect your family's health benefits. Under the Consolidated Omnibus Budget Reconciliation Act (COBRA), you, your covered spouse, and your dependent children may be eligible to purchase extended health coverage under your employer's plan if you lose your job, change employers, get divorced, or upon occurrence of certain other events. Coverage can range from 18 to 36 months depending on your situation. COBRA applies to most employers with 20 or more workers and requires your plan to notify you of your rights. Most plans require eligible individuals to make their COBRA election within 60 days of the plan's notice. Be sure to follow up with your plan sponsor if you don't receive notice, and make sure you respond within the allotted time.

7. HIPAA can also help if you are changing jobs, particularly if you have a medical condition. HIPAA generally limits pre-existing condition exclusions to a maximum of 12 months (18 months for late enrollees). HIPAA also requires this maximum period to be reduced by the length of time you had prior "creditable coverage." You should receive a certificate documenting your prior creditable coverage from your old plan when coverage ends.

8. Plan for retirement. Before you retire, find out what health benefits, if any, extend to you and your spouse during your retirement years. Consult with your employer's human resources office, your union, the plan administrator, and check your SPD. Make sure there is no conflicting information among these sources about the benefits your family will receive or the circumstances under which they can change or be eliminated. With this information in hand, you can make other important choices, like finding out if you are eligible for Medicare and Medigap insurance coverage.

9. Know how to file an appeal if a health benefits claim is denied. Understand how your plan handles grievances and where to make appeals of the plan's decisions. Keep records and copies of correspondence. Check your health benefits package and your SPD to determine who is responsible for handling problems with benefit claims. Contact PWBA for customer service assistance if you are unable to obtain a response to your complaint.

10. You can take steps to improve the quality of the healthcare and the health benefits your family receives. Look for and use things like Quality Reports and Accreditation Reports whenever you can. Quality reports may contain consumer ratings -- how satisfied consumers are with the doctors in their plan, for instance-- and clinical performance measures -- how well a healthcare organization prevents and treats illness. Accreditation reports provide information on how accredited organizations meet national standards, and often include clinical performance measures. Look for these quality measures whenever possible. Consult "Your Guide to Choosing Quality Health Care" on the Internet at **www.ahcpr.gov/consumer**.

Medicaid

Illness strikes both rich and poor families. For low-income families, Medicaid is available to defer the costs of treatment. In the following pages, you will learn the basics about Medicaid as well as useful contact information on how to find more in-depth information.

Medicaid is a joint federal and state program that helps pay medical costs for some people with low incomes and limited resources. Medicaid programs vary from state to state. You can find more information about Medicaid on the HCFA.gov Web site at **http://www.hcfa.gov/medicaid/medicaid.htm**.

NORD's Medication Assistance Programs

Finally, the National Organization for Rare Disorders, Inc. (NORD) administers medication programs sponsored by humanitarian-minded pharmaceutical and biotechnology companies to help uninsured or under-insured individuals secure life-saving or life-sustaining drugs.[39] NORD programs ensure that certain vital drugs are available "to those families whose income is too high to qualify for Medicaid but too low to pay for their prescribed medications." The program has standards for fairness, equity, and unbiased eligibility. It currently covers some 14 programs for nine pharmaceutical companies. NORD also offers early access programs for investigational new drugs (IND) under the approved "Treatment INDs" programs of the Food and Drug Administration (FDA). In these programs, a limited number of individuals can receive investigational drugs that have yet to be approved by the FDA. These programs are generally designed for rare medical conditions. For more information, visit **www.rarediseases.org**.

Additional Resources

In addition to the references already listed in this chapter, you may need more information on health insurance, hospitals, or the healthcare system in general. The NIH has set up an excellent guidance Web site that addresses these and other issues. Topics include:[40]

- Health Insurance:
  http://www.nlm.nih.gov/medlineplus/healthinsurance.html
- Health Statistics:
  http://www.nlm.nih.gov/medlineplus/healthstatistics.html
- HMO and Managed Care:
  http://www.nlm.nih.gov/medlineplus/managedcare.html
- Hospice Care: **http://www.nlm.nih.gov/medlineplus/hospicecare.html**
- Medicaid: **http://www.nlm.nih.gov/medlineplus/medicaid.html**
- Medicare: **http://www.nlm.nih.gov/medlineplus/medicare.html**
- Nursing Homes and Long-term Care:
  http://www.nlm.nih.gov/medlineplus/nursinghomes.html
- Patient's Rights, Confidentiality, Informed Consent, Ombudsman Programs, Privacy and Patient Issues:
  http://www.nlm.nih.gov/medlineplus/patientissues.html
- Veteran's Health, Persian Gulf War, Gulf War Syndrome, Agent Orange:
  http://www.nlm.nih.gov/medlineplus/veteranshealth.html

---

[39] Adapted from NORD: **http://www.rarediseases.org/cgi-bin/nord/progserv#patient?id=rPIzL9oD&mv_pc=30**.
[40] You can access this information at:
http://www.nlm.nih.gov/medlineplus/healthsystem.html.

Vocabulary Builder

Aorta: The main trunk of the systemic arteries. [NIH]

Bacteria: Unicellular prokaryotic microorganisms which generally possess rigid cell walls, multiply by cell division, and exhibit three principal forms: round or coccal, rodlike or bacillary, and spiral or spirochetal. [NIH]

Capsules: Hard or soft soluble containers used for the oral administration of medicine. [NIH]

Choline: A basic constituent of lecithin that is found in many plants and animal organs. It is important as a precursor of acetylcholine, as a methyl donor in various metabolic processes, and in lipid metabolism. [NIH]

Cyclodextrins: A homologous group of cyclic glucans consisting of alpha-1,4 bound glucose units obtained by the action of cyclodextrin glucanotransferase on starch or similar substrates. The enzyme is produced by certain species of Bacillus. Cyclodextrins form inclusion complexes with a wide variety of substances. [NIH]

Diarrhea: Passage of excessively liquid or excessively frequent stools. [NIH]

Hepatic: Pertaining to the liver. [EU]

Intestinal: Pertaining to the intestine. [EU]

Iodine: A nonmetallic element of the halogen group that is represented by the atomic symbol I, atomic number 53, and atomic weight of 126.90. It is a nutritionally essential element, especially important in thyroid hormone synthesis. In solution, it has anti-infective properties and is used topically. [NIH]

Melanoma: A tumour arising from the melanocytic system of the skin and other organs. When used alone the term refers to malignant melanoma. [EU]

Membranes: Thin layers of tissue which cover parts of the body, separate adjacent cavities, or connect adjacent structures. [NIH]

Morale: The prevailing temper or spirit of an individual or group in relation to the tasks or functions which are expected. [NIH]

Neonatology: A subspecialty of Pediatrics concerned with the newborn infant. [NIH]

Neurosurgery: A surgical specialty concerned with the treatment of diseases and disorders of the brain, spinal cord, and peripheral and sympathetic nervous system. [NIH]

Niacin: Water-soluble vitamin of the B complex occurring in various animal and plant tissues. Required by the body for the formation of coenzymes NAD and NADP. Has pellagra-curative, vasodilating, and antilipemic properties. [NIH]

Oxidation: The act of oxidizing or state of being oxidized. Chemically it consists in the increase of positive charges on an atom or the loss of negative charges. Most biological oxidations are accomplished by the removal of a pair of hydrogen atoms (dehydrogenation) from a molecule. Such oxidations must be accompanied by reduction of an acceptor molecule. Univalent o. indicates loss of one electron; divalent o., the loss of two electrons. [EU]

Photosensitization: The development of abnormally heightened reactivity of the skin to sunlight. [EU]

Potassium: An element that is in the alkali group of metals. It has an atomic symbol K, atomic number 19, and atomic weight 39.10. It is the chief cation in the intracellular fluid of muscle and other cells. Potassium ion is a strong electrolyte and it plays a significant role in the regulation of fluid volume and maintenance of the water-electrolyte balance. [NIH]

Proteoglycans: Glycoproteins which have a very high polysaccharide content. [NIH]

Riboflavin: Nutritional factor found in milk, eggs, malted barley, liver, kidney, heart, and leafy vegetables. The richest natural source is yeast. It occurs in the free form only in the retina of the eye, in whey, and in urine; its principal forms in tissues and cells are as FMN and FAD. [NIH]

Selenium: An element with the atomic symbol Se, atomic number 34, and atomic weight 78.96. It is an essential micronutrient for mammals and other animals but is toxic in large amounts. Selenium protects intracellular structures against oxidative damage. It is an essential component of glutathione peroxidase. [NIH]

Sphingomyelins: A class of sphingolipids found largely in the brain and other nervous tissue. They contain phosphocholine or phosphoethanolamine as their polar head group so therefore are the only sphingolipids classified as phospholipids. [NIH]

Thermoregulation: Heat regulation. [EU]

Thyroxine: An amino acid of the thyroid gland which exerts a stimulating effect on thyroid metabolism. [NIH]

Toxic: Pertaining to, due to, or of the nature of a poison or toxin; manifesting the symptoms of severe infection. [EU]

Viruses: Minute infectious agents whose genomes are composed of DNA or RNA, but not both. They are characterized by a lack of independent metabolism and the inability to replicate outside living host cells. [NIH]

ONLINE GLOSSARIES

The Internet provides access to a number of free-to-use medical dictionaries and glossaries. The National Library of Medicine has compiled the following list of online dictionaries:

- ADAM Medical Encyclopedia (A.D.A.M., Inc.), comprehensive medical reference: **http://www.nlm.nih.gov/medlineplus/encyclopedia.html**
- MedicineNet.com Medical Dictionary (MedicineNet, Inc.): **http://www.medterms.com/Script/Main/hp.asp**
- Merriam-Webster Medical Dictionary (Inteli-Health, Inc.): **http://www.intelihealth.com/IH/**
- Multilingual Glossary of Technical and Popular Medical Terms in Eight European Languages (European Commission) - Danish, Dutch, English, French, German, Italian, Portuguese, and Spanish: **http://allserv.rug.ac.be/~rvdstich/eugloss/welcome.html**
- On-line Medical Dictionary (CancerWEB): **http://www.graylab.ac.uk/omd/**
- Technology Glossary (National Library of Medicine) - Health Care Technology: **http://www.nlm.nih.gov/nichsr/ta101/ta10108.htm**
- Terms and Definitions (Office of Rare Diseases): **http://rarediseases.info.nih.gov/ord/glossary_a-e.html**

Beyond these, MEDLINEplus contains a very user-friendly encyclopedia covering every aspect of medicine (licensed from A.D.A.M., Inc.). The ADAM Medical Encyclopedia Web site address is **http://www.nlm.nih.gov/medlineplus/encyclopedia.html**. ADAM is also available on commercial Web sites such as drkoop.com (http://www.drkoop.com/) and Web MD (http://my.webmd.com/adam/asset/adam_disease_articles/a_to_z/a). Topics of interest can be researched by using keywords before continuing elsewhere, as these basic definitions and concepts will be useful in more advanced areas of research. You may choose to print various pages specifically relating to Niemann-Pick disease and keep them on file.

Online Dictionary Directories

The following are additional online directories compiled by the National Library of Medicine, including a number of specialized medical dictionaries and glossaries:

- Medical Dictionaries: Medical & Biological (World Health Organization):
  http://www.who.int/hlt/virtuallibrary/English/diction.htm#Medical
- MEL-Michigan Electronic Library List of Online Health and Medical Dictionaries (Michigan Electronic Library):
  http://mel.lib.mi.us/health/health-dictionaries.html
- Patient Education: Glossaries (DMOZ Open Directory Project):
  http://dmoz.org/Health/Education/Patient_Education/Glossaries/
- Web of Online Dictionaries (Bucknell University):
  http://www.yourdictionary.com/diction5.html#medicine

NIEMANN-PICK DISEASE GLOSSARY

The following is a complete glossary of terms used in this sourcebook. The definitions are derived from official public sources including the National Institutes of Health [NIH] and the European Union [EU]. After this glossary, we list a number of additional hardbound and electronic glossaries and dictionaries that you may wish to consult.

Aberrant: Wandering or deviating from the usual or normal course. [EU]

Adolescence: The period of life beginning with the appearance of secondary sex characteristics and terminating with the cessation of somatic growth. The years usually referred to as adolescence lie between 13 and 18 years of age. [NIH]

Aorta: The main trunk of the systemic arteries. [NIH]

Assay: Determination of the amount of a particular constituent of a mixture, or of the biological or pharmacological potency of a drug. [EU]

Ataxia: Failure of muscular coordination; irregularity of muscular action. [EU]

Bacteria: Unicellular prokaryotic microorganisms which generally possess rigid cell walls, multiply by cell division, and exhibit three principal forms: round or coccal, rodlike or bacillary, and spiral or spirochetal. [NIH]

Bile: An emulsifying agent produced in the liver and secreted into the duodenum. Its composition includes bile acids and salts, cholesterol, and electrolytes. It aids digestion of fats in the duodenum. [NIH]

Biliary: Pertaining to the bile, to the bile ducts, or to the gallbladder. [EU]

Biodegradation: The series of processes by which living systems render chemicals less noxious to the environment. [EU]

Biosynthesis: The building up of a chemical compound in the physiologic processes of a living organism. [EU]

Capsules: Hard or soft soluble containers used for the oral administration of medicine. [NIH]

Carbohydrate: An aldehyde or ketone derivative of a polyhydric alcohol, particularly of the pentahydric and hexahydric alcohols. They are so named because the hydrogen and oxygen are usually in the proportion to form water, $(CH_2O)_n$. The most important carbohydrates are the starches, sugars, celluloses, and gums. They are classified into mono-, di-, tri-, poly- and heterosaccharides. [EU]

Cardiovascular: Pertaining to the heart and blood vessels. [EU]

Cerebellar: Pertaining to the cerebellum. [EU]

Cerebellum: Part of the metencephalon that lies in the posterior cranial fossa behind the brain stem. It is concerned with the coordination of movement. [NIH]

Cholera: An acute diarrheal disease endemic in India and Southeast Asia whose causative agent is vibrio cholerae. This condition can lead to severe dehydration in a matter of hours unless quickly treated. [NIH]

Cholesterol: The principal sterol of all higher animals, distributed in body tissues, especially the brain and spinal cord, and in animal fats and oils. [NIH]

Choline: A basic constituent of lecithin that is found in many plants and animal organs. It is important as a precursor of acetylcholine, as a methyl donor in various metabolic processes, and in lipid metabolism. [NIH]

Chronic: Persisting over a long period of time. [EU]

Contraception: The prevention of conception or impregnation. [EU]

Contraceptive: An agent that diminishes the likelihood of or prevents conception. [EU]

Cortical: Pertaining to or of the nature of a cortex or bark. [EU]

Cyclodextrins: A homologous group of cyclic glucans consisting of alpha-1,4 bound glucose units obtained by the action of cyclodextrin glucanotransferase on starch or similar substrates. The enzyme is produced by certain species of Bacillus. Cyclodextrins form inclusion complexes with a wide variety of substances. [NIH]

Cytokines: Non-antibody proteins secreted by inflammatory leukocytes and some non-leukocytic cells, that act as intercellular mediators. They differ from classical hormones in that they are produced by a number of tissue or cell types rather than by specialized glands. They generally act locally in a paracrine or autocrine rather than endocrine manner. [NIH]

Dementia: An acquired organic mental disorder with loss of intellectual abilities of sufficient severity to interfere with social or occupational functioning. The dysfunction is multifaceted and involves memory, behavior, personality, judgment, attention, spatial relations, language, abstract thought, and other executive functions. The intellectual decline is usually progressive, and initially spares the level of consciousness. [NIH]

Dendritic: 1. branched like a tree. 2. pertaining to or possessing dendrites. [EU]

Diarrhea: Passage of excessively liquid or excessively frequent stools. [NIH]

Diffusion: The process of becoming diffused, or widely spread; the spontaneous movement of molecules or other particles in solution, owing to their random thermal motion, to reach a uniform concentration throughout the solvent, a process requiring no addition of energy to the system. [EU]

Drosophila: A genus of small, two-winged flies containing approximately 900 described species. These organisms are the most extensively studied of all genera from the standpoint of genetics and cytology. [NIH]

Dystonia: Disordered tonicity of muscle. [EU]

Electrophysiological: Pertaining to electrophysiology, that is a branch of physiology that is concerned with the electric phenomena associated with living bodies and involved in their functional activity. [EU]

Embryo: In animals, those derivatives of the fertilized ovum that eventually become the offspring, during their period of most rapid development, i.e., after the long axis appears until all major structures are represented. In man, the developing organism is an embryo from about two weeks after fertilization to the end of seventh or eighth week. [EU]

Empiric: Empirical; depending upon experience or observation alone, without using scientific method or theory. [EU]

Enzyme: A protein molecule that catalyses chemical reactions of other substances without itself being destroyed or altered upon completion of the reactions. Enzymes are classified according to the recommendations of the Nomenclature Committee of the International Union of Biochemistry. Each enzyme is assigned a recommended name and an Enzyme Commission (EC) number. They are divided into six main groups; oxidoreductases, transferases, hydrolases, lyases, isomerases, and ligases. [EU]

Excitation: An act of irritation or stimulation or of responding to a stimulus; the addition of energy, as the excitation of a molecule by absorption of photons. [EU]

Exogenous: Developed or originating outside the organism, as exogenous disease. [EU]

Extracellular: Outside a cell or cells. [EU]

Fibroblasts: Connective tissue cells which secrete an extracellular matrix rich in collagen and other macromolecules. [NIH]

Genotype: The genetic constitution of the individual; the characterization of the genes. [NIH]

Glucose: D-glucose, a monosaccharide (hexose), $C_6H_{12}O_6$, also known as dextrose (q.v.), found in certain foodstuffs, especially fruits, and in the normal blood of all animals. It is the end product of carbohydrate metabolism and is the chief source of energy for living organisms, its utilization being controlled by insulin. Excess glucose is converted to glycogen and stored in the liver and muscles for use as needed and, beyond that, is converted to fat and stored as adipose tissue. Glucose appears in the urine in diabetes mellitus. [EU]

Gonads: The gamete-producing glands, ovary or testis. [NIH]

Hematology: A subspecialty of internal medicine concerned with morphology, physiology, and pathology of the blood and blood-forming tissues. [NIH]

Hepatic: Pertaining to the liver. [EU]

Hepatitis: Inflammation of the liver. [EU]

Homeostasis: A tendency to stability in the normal body states (internal environment) of the organism. It is achieved by a system of control mechanisms activated by negative feedback; e.g. a high level of carbon dioxide in extracellular fluid triggers increased pulmonary ventilation, which in turn causes a decrease in carbon dioxide concentration. [EU]

Hormones: Chemical substances having a specific regulatory effect on the activity of a certain organ or organs. The term was originally applied to substances secreted by various endocrine glands and transported in the bloodstream to the target organs. It is sometimes extended to include those substances that are not produced by the endocrine glands but that have similar effects. [NIH]

Hybridization: The genetic process of crossbreeding to produce a hybrid. Hybrid nucleic acids can be formed by nucleic acid hybridization of DNA and RNA molecules. Protein hybridization allows for hybrid proteins to be formed from polypeptide chains. [NIH]

Hydrophilic: Readily absorbing moisture; hygroscopic; having strongly polar groups that readily interact with water. [EU]

Hyperlipidemia: An excess of lipids in the blood. [NIH]

Immunohistochemistry: Histochemical localization of immunoreactive substances using labeled antibodies as reagents. [NIH]

Implantation: The insertion or grafting into the body of biological, living, inert, or radioactive material. [EU]

Infiltration: The diffusion or accumulation in a tissue or cells of substances not normal to it or in amounts of the normal. Also, the material so accumulated. [EU]

Insulin: A protein hormone secreted by beta cells of the pancreas. Insulin plays a major role in the regulation of glucose metabolism, generally promoting the cellular utilization of glucose. It is also an important regulator of protein and lipid metabolism. Insulin is used as a drug to control insulin-dependent diabetes mellitus. [NIH]

Intestinal: Pertaining to the intestine. [EU]

Invasive: 1. having the quality of invasiveness. 2. involving puncture or incision of the skin or insertion of an instrument or foreign material into the body; said of diagnostic techniques. [EU]

Iodine: A nonmetallic element of the halogen group that is represented by the atomic symbol I, atomic number 53, and atomic weight of 126.90. It is a nutritionally essential element, especially important in thyroid hormone synthesis. In solution, it has anti-infective properties and is used topically. [NIH]

Kinetic: Pertaining to or producing motion. [EU]

Lesion: Any pathological or traumatic discontinuity of tissue or loss of function of a part. [EU]

Ligation: Application of a ligature to tie a vessel or strangulate a part. [NIH]

Lipid: Any of a heterogeneous group of flats and fatlike substances characterized by being water-insoluble and being extractable by nonpolar (or fat) solvents such as alcohol, ether, chloroform, benzene, etc. All contain as a major constituent aliphatic hydrocarbons. The lipids, which are easily stored in the body, serve as a source of fuel, are an important constituent of cell structure, and serve other biological functions. Lipids may be considered to include fatty acids, neutral fats, waxes, and steroids. Compound lipids comprise the glycolipids, lipoproteins, and phospholipids. [EU]

Lipoprotein: Any of the lipid-protein complexes in which lipids are transported in the blood; lipoprotein particles consist of a spherical hydrophobic core of triglycerides or cholesterol esters surrounded by an amphipathic monolayer of phospholipids, cholesterol, and apolipoproteins; the four principal classes are high-density, low-density, and very-low-density lipoproteins and chylomicrons. [EU]

Localization: 1. the determination of the site or place of any process or lesion. 2. restriction to a circumscribed or limited area. 3. prelocalization. [EU]

Malformation: A morphologic defect resulting from an intrinsically abnormal developmental process. [EU]

Melanoma: A tumour arising from the melanocytic system of the skin and other organs. When used alone the term refers to malignant melanoma. [EU]

Membrane: A thin layer of tissue which covers a surface, lines a cavity or divides a space or organ. [EU]

Microscopy: The application of microscope magnification to the study of materials that cannot be properly seen by the unaided eye. [NIH]

Molecular: Of, pertaining to, or composed of molecules : a very small mass of matter. [EU]

Morale: The prevailing temper or spirit of an individual or group in relation to the tasks or functions which are expected. [NIH]

Neonatal: Pertaining to the first four weeks after birth. [EU]

Neonatology: A subspecialty of Pediatrics concerned with the newborn infant. [NIH]

Neuroanatomy: Study of the anatomy of the nervous system as a specialty or discipline. [NIH]

Neurology: A medical specialty concerned with the study of the structures, functions, and diseases of the nervous system. [NIH]

Neuronal: Pertaining to a neuron or neurons (= conducting cells of the nervous system). [EU]

Neurons: The basic cellular units of nervous tissue. Each neuron consists of a body, an axon, and dendrites. Their purpose is to receive, conduct, and transmit impulses in the nervous system. [NIH]

Neurosurgery: A surgical specialty concerned with the treatment of diseases and disorders of the brain, spinal cord, and peripheral and sympathetic nervous system. [NIH]

Niacin: Water-soluble vitamin of the B complex occurring in various animal and plant tissues. Required by the body for the formation of coenzymes NAD and NADP. Has pellagra-curative, vasodilating, and antilipemic properties. [NIH]

Nickel: Nickel. A trace element with the atomic symbol Ni, atomic number 28, and atomic weight 58.69. It is a cofactor of the enzyme urease. [NIH]

Organelles: Specific particles of membrane-bound organized living substances present in eukaryotic cells, such as the mitochondria; the golgi apparatus; endoplasmic reticulum; lysomomes; plastids; and vacuoles. [NIH]

Ossicle: A small bone. [EU]

Otitis: Inflammation of the ear, which may be marked by pain, fever, abnormalities of hearing, hearing loss, tinnitus, and vertigo. [EU]

Ovary: Either of the paired glands in the female that produce the female germ cells and secrete some of the female sex hormones. [NIH]

Overdose: 1. to administer an excessive dose. 2. an excessive dose. [EU]

Oxidation: The act of oxidizing or state of being oxidized. Chemically it consists in the increase of positive charges on an atom or the loss of negative charges. Most biological oxidations are accomplished by the removal of a pair of hydrogen atoms (dehydrogenation) from a molecule. Such oxidations must be accompanied by reduction of an acceptor molecule. Univalent o. indicates loss of one electron; divalent o., the loss of two electrons. [EU]

Parkinsonism: A group of neurological disorders characterized by hypokinesia, tremor, and muscular rigidity. [EU]

Pediatrics: A medical specialty concerned with maintaining health and providing medical care to children from birth to adolescence. [NIH]

Pharmacokinetics: The action of drugs in the body over a period of time, including the processes of absorption, distribution, localization in tissues, biotransformation, and excretion. [EU]

Phenotype: The outward appearance of the individual. It is the product of interactions between genes and between the genotype and the environment. This includes the killer phenotype, characteristic of yeasts. [NIH]

Photosensitization: The development of abnormally heightened reactivity of the skin to sunlight. [EU]

Polypeptide: A peptide which on hydrolysis yields more than two amino acids; called tripeptides, tetrapeptides, etc. according to the number of amino acids contained. [EU]

Potassium: An element that is in the alkali group of metals. It has an atomic symbol K, atomic number 19, and atomic weight 39.10. It is the chief cation in the intracellular fluid of muscle and other cells. Potassium ion is a strong electrolyte and it plays a significant role in the regulation of fluid volume and maintenance of the water-electrolyte balance. [NIH]

Prenatal: Existing or occurring before birth, with reference to the fetus. [EU]

Presynaptic: Situated proximal to a synapse, or occurring before the synapse is crossed. [EU]

Prevalence: The total number of cases of a given disease in a specified population at a designated time. It is differentiated from incidence, which refers to the number of new cases in the population at a given time. [NIH]

Progressive: Advancing; going forward; going from bad to worse; increasing in scope or severity. [EU]

Proteins: Polymers of amino acids linked by peptide bonds. The specific sequence of amino acids determines the shape and function of the protein. [NIH]

Proteoglycans: Glycoproteins which have a very high polysaccharide content. [NIH]

Psychiatric: Pertaining to or within the purview of psychiatry. [EU]

Puberty: The period during which the secondary sex characteristics begin to develop and the capability of sexual reproduction is attained. [EU]

Pulmonary: Pertaining to the lungs. [EU]

Receptor: 1. a molecular structure within a cell or on the surface characterized by (1) selective binding of a specific substance and (2) a specific physiologic effect that accompanies the binding, e.g., cell-surface receptors for peptide hormones, neurotransmitters, antigens, complement fragments, and immunoglobulins and cytoplasmic receptors for steroid hormones. 2. a sensory nerve terminal that responds to stimuli of various kinds. [EU]

Recombinant: 1. a cell or an individual with a new combination of genes not found together in either parent; usually applied to linked genes. [EU]

Retrograde: 1. moving backward or against the usual direction of flow. 2. degenerating, deteriorating, or catabolic. [EU]

Riboflavin: Nutritional factor found in milk, eggs, malted barley, liver, kidney, heart, and leafy vegetables. The richest natural source is yeast. It occurs in the free form only in the retina of the eye, in whey, and in urine; its principal forms in tissues and cells are as FMN and FAD. [NIH]

Saccharomyces: A genus of ascomycetous fungi of the family Saccharomycetaceae, order saccharomycetales. [NIH]

Selenium: An element with the atomic symbol Se, atomic number 34, and atomic weight 78.96. It is an essential micronutrient for mammals and other animals but is toxic in large amounts. Selenium protects intracellular structures against oxidative damage. It is an essential component of glutathione peroxidase. [NIH]

Serum: The clear portion of any body fluid; the clear fluid moistening serous membranes. 2. blood serum; the clear liquid that separates from blood on clotting. 3. immune serum; blood serum from an immunized animal used for passive immunization; an antiserum; antitoxin, or antivenin. [EU]

Spectrum: A charted band of wavelengths of electromagnetic vibrations obtained by refraction and diffraction. By extension, a measurable range of activity, such as the range of bacteria affected by an antibiotic (antibacterial s.) or the complete range of manifestations of a disease. [EU]

Sphingomyelins: A class of sphingolipids found largely in the brain and other nervous tissue. They contain phosphocholine or phosphoethanolamine as their polar head group so therefore are the only sphingolipids classified as phospholipids. [NIH]

Sporadic: Neither endemic nor epidemic; occurring occasionally in a random or isolated manner. [EU]

Substrate: A substance upon which an enzyme acts. [EU]

Synaptic: Pertaining to or affecting a synapse (= site of functional apposition between neurons, at which an impulse is transmitted from one neuron to another by electrical or chemical means); pertaining to synapsis (= pairing off in point-for-point association of homologous chromosomes from the male and female pronuclei during the early prophase of meiosis). [EU]

Systemic: Pertaining to or affecting the body as a whole. [EU]

Thermoregulation: Heat regulation. [EU]

Thyroxine: An amino acid of the thyroid gland which exerts a stimulating effect on thyroid metabolism. [NIH]

Tone: 1. the normal degree of vigour and tension; in muscle, the resistance to passive elongation or stretch; tonus. 2. a particular quality of sound or of voice. 3. to make permanent, or to change, the colour of silver stain by chemical treatment, usually with a heavy metal. [EU]

Toxic: Pertaining to, due to, or of the nature of a poison or toxin; manifesting the symptoms of severe infection. [EU]

Toxin: A poison; frequently used to refer specifically to a protein produced by some higher plants, certain animals, and pathogenic bacteria, which is highly toxic for other living organisms. Such substances are differentiated from the simple chemical poisons and the vegetable alkaloids by their high molecular weight and antigenicity. [EU]

Transfusion: The introduction of whole blood or blood component directly into the blood stream. [EU]

Transplantation: The grafting of tissues taken from the patient's own body or from another. [EU]

Vestibular: Pertaining to or toward a vestibule. In dental anatomy, used to refer to the tooth surface directed toward the vestibule of the mouth. [EU]

Viruses: Minute infectious agents whose genomes are composed of DNA or RNA, but not both. They are characterized by a lack of independent metabolism and the inability to replicate outside living host cells. [NIH]

General Dictionaries and Glossaries

While the above glossary is essentially complete, the dictionaries listed here cover virtually all aspects of medicine, from basic words and phrases to more advanced terms (sorted alphabetically by title; hyperlinks provide rankings, information and reviews at Amazon.com):

- **Dictionary of Medical Acronymns & Abbreviations** by Stanley Jablonski (Editor), Paperback, 4th edition (2001), Lippincott Williams & Wilkins Publishers, ISBN: 1560534605,
  http://www.amazon.com/exec/obidos/ASIN/1560534605/icongroupinterna

- **Dictionary of Medical Terms : For the Nonmedical Person (Dictionary of Medical Terms for the Nonmedical Person, Ed 4)** by Mikel A. Rothenberg, M.D, et al, Paperback - 544 pages, 4th edition (2000), Barrons Educational Series, ISBN: 0764112015,
  http://www.amazon.com/exec/obidos/ASIN/0764112015/icongroupinterna

- **A Dictionary of the History of Medicine** by A. Sebastian, CD-Rom edition (2001), CRC Press-Parthenon Publishers, ISBN: 185070368X,
  http://www.amazon.com/exec/obidos/ASIN/185070368X/icongroupinterna

- **Dorland's Illustrated Medical Dictionary (Standard Version)** by Dorland, et al, Hardcover - 2088 pages, 29th edition (2000), W B Saunders Co, ISBN: 0721662544,
http://www.amazon.com/exec/obidos/ASIN/0721662544/icongroupinterna
- **Dorland's Electronic Medical Dictionary** by Dorland, et al, Software, 29th Book & CD-Rom edition (2000), Harcourt Health Sciences, ISBN: 0721694934,
http://www.amazon.com/exec/obidos/ASIN/0721694934/icongroupinterna
- **Dorland's Pocket Medical Dictionary (Dorland's Pocket Medical Dictionary, 26th Ed)** Hardcover - 912 pages, 26th edition (2001), W B Saunders Co, ISBN: 0721682812,
http://www.amazon.com/exec/obidos/ASIN/0721682812/icongroupinterna
/103-4193558-7304618
- **Melloni's Illustrated Medical Dictionary (Melloni's Illustrated Medical Dictionary, 4th Ed)** by Melloni, Hardcover, 4th edition (2001), CRC Press-Parthenon Publishers, ISBN: 85070094X,
http://www.amazon.com/exec/obidos/ASIN/85070094X/icongroupinterna
- **Stedman's Electronic Medical Dictionary Version 5.0 (CD-ROM for Windows and Macintosh, Individual)** by Stedmans, CD-ROM edition (2000), Lippincott Williams & Wilkins Publishers, ISBN: 0781726328,
http://www.amazon.com/exec/obidos/ASIN/0781726328/icongroupinterna
- **Stedman's Medical Dictionary** by Thomas Lathrop Stedman, Hardcover - 2098 pages, 27th edition (2000), Lippincott, Williams & Wilkins, ISBN: 068340007X,
http://www.amazon.com/exec/obidos/ASIN/068340007X/icongroupinterna
- **Tabers Cyclopedic Medical Dictionary (Thumb Index)** by Donald Venes (Editor), et al, Hardcover - 2439 pages, 19th edition (2001), F A Davis Co, ISBN: 0803606540,
http://www.amazon.com/exec/obidos/ASIN/0803606540/icongroupinterna

INDEX

A
Aberrant 45
Adolescence 18, 28, 64, 115, 120
Aorta 89
Assay 44, 49, 56, 58
Ataxia 18, 55

B
Bacteria 65, 82, 122, 123
Bile 28, 45, 115
Biliary 19
Biodegradation..................................11

C
Capsules 85
Carbohydrate......................40, 50, 84, 117
Cardiovascular 46
Cerebellar 48
Cerebellum 57, 61, 88, 116
Cholera 59
Cholesterol ... 11, 18, 21, 44, 45, 46, 48, 53, 55, 56, 59, 60, 63, 82, 84, 88, 90, 119
Choline 90
Chronic 50, 90, 102
Cortical 52
Cytokines 47

D
Dementia...51
Dendritic 52
Diarrhea 82
Diffusion 56, 63, 118

E
Electrophysiological 58
Embryo 62, 117
Empiric 54
Enzyme..... 11, 16, 49, 54, 63, 65, 110, 116, 117, 120, 122
Excitation 52, 62, 117
Exogenous 48, 62, 117

F
Fibroblasts.........................46, 48, 53, 87, 88

G
Genotype 54, 64, 121
Glucose 34, 40, 63, 110, 116, 117, 118
Gonads 52

H
Hepatic..90
Hepatitis 19
Homeostasis 45, 46
Hormones 52, 61, 64, 116, 120, 121
Hybridization 57
Hydrophilic 53
Hyperlipidemia 54

I
Implantation 49
Infiltration 47
Insulin..........................40, 48, 63, 117, 118
Intestinal 82
Invasive 55

L
Lesion 63, 119
Lipid 11, 20, 44, 48, 56, 58, 63, 110, 116, 118, 119
Lipoprotein 45, 59, 63, 119
Localization 56, 62, 64, 118, 120

M
Malformation 50
Melanoma 87, 110, 119
Membrane ... 11, 45, 46, 53, 56, 63, 87, 120
Microscopy 45, 53
Molecular 18, 44, 52, 55, 58, 64, 65, 121, 123

N
Neonatal 19
Neurons 47, 51, 56, 63, 65, 120, 122
Niacin 83

O
Ossicle...50
Otitis..50
Ovary 45
Overdose 83
Oxidation 89

P
Parkinsonism 51
Pharmacokinetics............................54
Phenotype 44, 52, 53, 54, 64, 121
Polypeptide 53, 62, 118
Potassium 84
Prenatal 23
Presynaptic 57
Prevalence 44, 58
Progressive 11, 18, 45, 50, 55, 57, 61, 110
Proteins ..44, 45, 46, 48, 57, 61, 62, 82, 84, 116, 118
Proteoglycans 89
Puberty 54, 55
Pulmonary 11, 54, 62, 118

R
Receptor........................... 48, 49, 57
Recombinant 54
Retrograde 44
Riboflavin..82

S
Selenium 84
Serum 65, 122
Spectrum 54
Sphingomyelins 87
Substrate 50
Synaptic 57
Systemic 110, 115

T
Thermoregulation 82
Thyroxine 84
Toxic 65, 83, 111, 122, 123
Toxin 59, 111, 123
Transplantation 11, 48, 54

V
Vestibular 50
Viruses 89

130 Niemann-Pick Disease

Printed in the United Kingdom
by Lightning Source UK Ltd.
126603UK00001B/43/A